I am thrilled and heartened by Dr. Crook's unique work. This collection of testimonials—real stories by real people who have unraveled and overcome the often insidious and confounding symptoms of yeast-related illness—has a powerful potential to heal. Each story is a key that unlocks the same door—the one to health.

—Beth Salmon, Editor in Chief, *Let's Live* magazine, "America's Foremost Health and Preventive Medicine Magazine."

To Michelle Hardee

With warm regards

William G (Billy) Crook

YEAST CONNECTION SUCCESS STORIES

A COLLECTION OF STORIES FROM PEOPLE WHO ARE WINNING THE BATTLE AGAINST DEVASTATING ILLNESS

BY
WILLIAM G. CROOK, M.D.

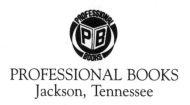

PROFESSIONAL BOOKS
Jackson, Tennessee

▪ DISCLAIMER ▪

This book describes relationships that have been observed between the common yeast germ *Candida albicans* and health problems that affect people of all ages and both sexes—especially premenopausal women. *I have written it to serve only as a general informational guide and reference source for both professionals and nonprofessionals.*

For obvious reasons I cannot assume the medical or legal responsibility of having the contents of this book considered as a prescription for anyone.

Treatment of health disorders, including those which appear to be yeast connected, must be supervised by a physician or other licensed health professional. Accordingly, you and the professional who examines and treats you must take the responsibility for the uses made of this book.

Table of Contents

Section Three: Women (Over 50)

Section Four: Teens/Children

Dedication

I would like to dedicate this book to John Adams. I met this Nashville, Tennessee typesetter and his wife, Carol, in early 1983 as I worked to put together the first hardback edition of *The Yeast Connection*. Since that time, he and his small staff have typeset each of the books I've written.

John has not only carried out his work in a superb, professional manner, he's also served as a consultant and editor in many different ways. He styled the books, advised me and my staff how to divide them, put them together, where and how to place illustrations and much, much more. During all this work together, I met with him in his offices in and around Nashville. He's also met me and members of my staff at a restaurant halfway between Nashville and Jackson.

His suggestions and recommendations have been firm, comprehensive and varied. Although I argued with him at times, I'd usually find out that he was right. He's also served as a kind, kind friend and in October 1998, about three days after I underwent a total surgical replacement of my left knee, John and Carol drove the 400 plus miles round trip to see me in a Memphis hospital. John is a courageous, talented, Tennessee "good ol' boy" with a wonderful sense of humor. I treasure John as a true friend whose work may often go unrecognized.

Acknowledgments

To Janet Gregory. This book was conceived by Janet, who has worked for and with me for about 18 years—part-time and full-time. She's always done her work quietly, efficiently and with amazing skill and speed.

Although she began in the days before computers, and as far as I know took no special training, she has mastered technique and skills which I still don't understand or comprehend—like using a scanner, retrieving e-mail messages, searching the web and printing out pages of information.

I stand back in amazement, awe and admiration as I look at the work this quiet, shy, talented, efficient, single mother of a 15-year-old daughter turns out each week that she works with me.

There are countless other people who have helped me along the way during my yeast connection journey. Included are my patients, people who have written letters and sent me messages by fax or e-mail. Also, physicians, nurses and many other professionals. All have taught me many things that I did not know and would not have known if they had not helped me.

I'm grateful to the people who shared their stories included in this book and to three other members of my small staff, Brenda Harris, Jan Torre and Georgia Deaton. Their advice, help and skills of various sorts helped make this book possible.

Finally, thanks to Betsy, the wonderful girl I married almost 59 years ago. She's had to listen to my thousands of words even though many times she wished I were taking her out to dinner, to a movie or watching a TV sitcom with her.

Foreword

This book is a message to you. Its messenger, Dr. William G. Crook, combines clinical experience, passion, truth, simple humanity and humility as much as any medical author of our time. The truth he speaks comes from the stories of people like you. They are people who have something important to tell all of us about our options for solving puzzles of chronic health problems that range from persistent itchy ear canals to devastating depression, malaise, and fatigue. The stories are important because they truly tell of individual success in overcoming illness.

Perhaps more important is that the stories are not about a particular disease or diagnosis. They are about a common and current epidemic that affects different people in very different ways. Suppose you have something bad wrong with you—an ongoing disturbance of your breathing, digestion, skin, hormones, ability to concentrate; or fatigue, pain, or itching.

You try waiting, hope and denial, but this time they don't work. You try over-the-counter drugs and then prescription drugs. They don't work, and they cause side effects. Then you try a yeast-free diet and nystatin for three weeks and it works. You are delighted. You want to tell the world, starting with your doctor. She shrugs and rolls her eyes saying, "I have not seen any credible scientific evidence (shrug) that your condition would have anything to do with this so-called yeast problem (eye-roll), which is unproven." End of story.

Stories have an uphill fight. There is an official way for stories to find their way into the fabric of accepted medical Truth. First the description of a person's story is stripped of information not required to place it into a diagnostic category, and it is pooled with other stories. Then all concerned are divided into like *groups* and given one of two or more treatments for the condition. Analysis of the data produced in a prospective double-blind placebo-controlled study may reveal a difference between the groups of individuals signifying a response to treatment for the *condition* that would not have occurred by chance alone.

Many participants would have responded to the placebo (inert substance disguised to look real). Many others would have failed to respond to the real medicine. The treatment is, however, proven for the condition. It has to do with groups of people and the condition that is defined by their similarities. It takes lots of money, a long time, and may take some lives.

For example, in 1975 some doctors showed that a supplement of the B-vitamin, folic acid, could prevent certain serious birth defects. Before that every doctor in the world could shrug and eye-roll in response to a question about this connection. A prudent consumer or her physician, weighing the new 1975 evidence, could have made a *private health* decision to supplement folic acid. The *public health* policy that women ought to supplement folic acid waited twenty years while millions of dollars were spent on research studies in which women given placebos gave birth to defective babies.

We pay a necessarily high price for public health policy. Private health policy— the personal options you may wish to consider after the failure of hope and denial— is not cheap either, but it is your call. You pay for it with the time and effort to explore the options that have brought success to others like you. Not like you so much in terms of old-fashioned diagnostic categories. More like you in terms of new ways of thinking about your personal illness—not as a victim of the attack of a disease, but as an individual in whom the tip of some crucial balance has lowered your threshold for feeling sick.

Individuals living in North America since 1960 should be aware of three factors that tip the balance for many people in many diagnostic categories: too little magnesium or omega-3 fatty acids and too much of a common intestinal microbe from the large family of germs known collectively as yeasts.

Dr. Crook's stories focus on the yeast problem, which results when antibiotics injure your body's most vulnerable organ: the population of germs inhabiting the digestive tract. His previous books have made him the center of a polarized debate that began in 1977 when Dr. Orian Truss of Birmingham, Alabama first presented stories of patients who exemplified the mischief yeast problems can do. Dr. Truss's observations were denied and his "theory" was criticized, opposed, denounced, discredited, and "disproved" with all the haste, vehemence and carelessness mainstream medicine reserves for its heretics.

Into this fray came Dr. Crook. He seemed to confuse retirement age with a signal to put a bear hug on a new body of knowledge and squeeze it with all the might, persistence, and love he had already poured into his first career as a practicing physician. Not an ordinary physician. One who took equally into his heart the teaching of his professors from the best teaching centers and the lessons learned from listening to his patients for two generations.

He learned to navigate the gap—some would say the abyss— between the proofs of the ivory tower and the truths of everyday practice. He has lived, thrived, and triumphed in that gap by being a patient listener, a voluminous correspondent, determined teacher, and a generous friend to his patients and his colleagues. In this book he gives you the message of lessons he has learned as the student of his patients and the hundreds of people who have corresponded with him. These are lessons that will teach you respect. Respect for individuality in its infinite expressions. Respect for the power of an individual story to expand your private health options. Respect for your own grasp on your medical decisions. And respect for Billy Crook, a great physician, listener, and teller of stories.

Sidney MacDonald Baker, MD
Weston, CT
September 2001

Introduction

Since my first yeast book, *The Yeast Connection,** was published in hardback in 1983, I've received over 90,000 phone calls, letters, faxes and e-mail messages. Countless numbers of them have come from people who have searched in vain for a physician interested in yeast-related problems.

Because of this torrent of requests, with the help of friends and relatives, the International Health Foundation (IHF)† was established in 1985 to help me respond. Then, after receiving its charter from the state of Tennessee, the Internal Revenue Service classified IHF as a 501(c)3 organization. As the years went by, I continued to receive letters, including many which have made me smile and even glow. Here's the first sentence of one of these letters.

Dr. Crook, I love you! Your books and IHF saved my life. Without this information and help I don't know where I'd be. Probably in a mental hospital or a cemetery.

---

*I do not recommend this "classic" book because it's *out of date*—only ten pages have been changed in the 400-page 1986 paperback edition. My most recent yeast publications, which you'll find in most health food stores and some bookstores are *The Yeast Connection Handbook*, *The Yeast Connection Cookbook* and *Tired—So Tired! and the "yeast connection."*

†This tiny foundation with three part-time staff members continues to try to provide help for people who write and call. Please look at the IHF section on my website, www.candida-yeast.com.

In many of these letters people told me wonderful stories of how they had regained their health and their lives by following a comprehensive treatment program which enabled them to conquer the yeast "beast."

As you read these stories, you'll see that most people told of their "ups and downs." Here's why. Taking antiyeast medication and making dietary changes does not provide a "quick fix" or a cure for fatigue, headache, depression or other symptoms.

It is only when your immune system becomes weakened because of repeated use of antibiotic drugs, exposure to environmental chemicals, nutritionally deficient diets and other causes that candida yeasts multiply and make you sick. Here are excerpts of the comments of Dr. George Kroker which I included in my 700-page 1995 book, *The Yeast Connection and the Woman.*

I'm writing in response to your request for my impressions in treating Candida Related Complex (CRC). As you know, I'm a university-trained, board-certified physician. I treated my first patient with this illness in 1978 . . . I became intrigued as to why this illness had such diverse manifestations. As you know, I subsequently reviewed the classical literature on candida-related pathology and contributed a chapter on this subject to an allergy textbook. I've treated several thousand patients with this illness over the last 14 years.* I've arrived at the following clinical impressions over that time.

---

*Dr. Kroker has seen many more patients with these problems in the seven years since he sent me this message.

1. *Candida Related Complex (CRC) cannot be treated successfully without simultaneous attention to a sugar and yeast-free diet.*
2. *CRC often is associated with other illnesses, most notably mold allergy, chemical sensitivities, autoimmune thyroiditis, and food intolerances. Unless these illnesses are screened for, the treatment for candida may completely fail to ameliorate the patient's symptoms. I cannot overemphasize the 'total load' in dealing with these patients. This makes it hard to set up a study.*
3. *CRC seems to be a chronic and relapsing illness in many patients. They may have a remission and require no antifungal medication and be more lenient on their diet, only to relapse and have a return to illness with stress, dietary overindulgence, antibiotics, etc. CRC seems to co-exist frequently in patients with premenstrual syndrome and also in patients with chronic fatigue syndrome. Treating candida illness seems to often improve both of these other problems.*
4. *Unfortunately, candida remains a disease in search of a laboratory test for diagnosis. The best test remains the history and a one-month trial of antifungal medication and diet. I've tried to utilize antibody assays, cultures and ETC, and they all fall short of diagnostic certainty.*

Dr. Kroker is a superb physician and my good friend. I could write pages about him. Here are a few of the highlights.

I've called him and picked his brain many, many times.

◇ He and his wife, Leslie Peickert-Kroker, BSN, MS, wrote the Foreword to my 1989 book, *The Yeast Connection Cookbook* (co-authored by Marjorie Hurt Jones, R.N.).

◇ He serves as an active and generous contributing member of the Advisory Board of the International Health Foundation.

◇ He wrote the Foreword to *The Yeast Connection Handbook.*

I only wish that there were thousands of physicians in the U.S. (and in the world) like George F. Kroker, M.D., FACAI, FAAEM.

Now then. There are hundreds of families of yeasts and molds. Some are friendly and some are not—and some are sort of "in between." One of these "in between" yeasts—*Candida albicans*—normally lives on the inner warm membranes of your body. It causes no trouble when your immune system is strong. But when you take antibiotics—especially a lot of them—or high sugar diets, candida yeasts multiply. Birth control pills also encourage the growth of these yeasts. *Candida albicans* lives *especially* in the digestive tract of people of both sexes, and in the vagina in women. Candida and other fungi may also multiply on your respiratory membranes (nose, sinuses and lungs), especially if you've taken many antibiotics or oral, injected or inhaled steroids. Although *Candida albicans* is well known for the problems it causes in the vagina, most physicians don't seem to be aware of the problems it causes in many, many parts of the body.

The relationship of candida to headache, fatigue, depression and other generalized symptoms was first reported by C. Orian Truss, M.D., a Birmingham, Alabama internist and allergist. This brilliant pioneer physician also reported that recurrent ear problems and behavior and learning problems in children may be related to candida. He also noted that multiple sclerosis, sexual dysfunction and many other disorders were candida related.

Dr. Truss first reported his findings in a small Canadian medical journal (*The Journal of Orthomolecular Psychiatry*) in the late 70s and early 80s and in a book, *The Missing Diagnosis.** Word of his observations spread to the public in an article in *Atlanta Magazine* which was re-published in the Holiday Inn magazine, *Inn America*. Truss' observations were also featured on a popular one-hour CNN program, *The Freeman Report*.

In 1979 I learned from a patient how yeasts make people sick, and I began to use the Truss regimen on some of my difficult patients. *His observations changed my practice and my life.* I hadn't thought about writing a book on this subject until I appeared on a regional TV program, WLW-TV in Cincinnati (January 1983). Following a 15-minute back and forth discussion with my host, Bob Braun, my mailbox was swamped with requests for information—over 7300 letters in one week.

This amazing response prompted me to push aside another book I was working on and write *The Yeast Connection* which I self-published in hardback in December 1983. A revised and expanded paperback edition of this book was co-published by my company, Professionals Books, and Vin-

*To obtain information about this book, write to The Missing Diagnosis, Box 26508, Birmingham, AL 35226.

tage/Random House in October 1986. Since then I've written eight other books which include a discussion of the role candida yeasts play in making many people sick.

I hope you'll enjoy reading the stories in this book as much as I have. If you have a yeast connection success story you'd like to share with me, I'd love to receive it.

William G. "Billy" Crook, M.D.

SECTION ONE

Women in Their 20s and 30s

Harriet*

My life had turned into a nightmare. I pleaded to doctors for help but they didn't have a clue to what was wrong with me. Every test they ran came out normal. I had been suffering for years with ulcerative colitis and panic attacks, but now it had gotten worse.

After several rounds of antibiotics, I started having depression and anxiety so bad that I stopped attending social events. I would burst into tears for no reason. This went along with alternating fatigue and bursts of energy, blood sugar drops, irritability and mood swings. Then my esophagus and stomach became inflamed and a strange rash broke out on my legs.

Finally, my doctor told me about Dr. Crook's book. Maybe I could find some answers there. I did just as he prescribed and read the book. This book was describing me. How could he know me so well?

I was on a low-carbohydrate diet already, so I made a phone call to my doctor to try out a medicine called nystatin. This antifungal prescription, taken as directed, slowly started to change my life. I combined it with a yeast-free diet. All my stomach symptoms, my depression and anxiety left, and so did my fatigue.

---

*Not her real name.

Thank you Dr. Crook. You'll never know how happy you've made many people like me. Keep on going and never become discouraged.

✦✦✦ ✉ ✦✦✦

Harriet, an attractive young woman in her late 20s that I did not know, walked into my office with her mother in early 2001 and brought me this wonderful story. It made my day, my week and my month!

Dr. Crook

Jamie

I was a healthy child until I was about 8. Then I got a sore throat and the doctors put me on antibiotics. From what my mother tells me, I'd get one infection and then another. They would always give me antibiotics. I took them for 210 days in a year and a half. During that time, I was hospitalized four times and given all sorts of tests and many different medications.

Comment by Dr. Crook: Here are excerpts from a letter her mother, Sandy, sent me about 14 years ago.

Jamie's health problems continued on through 1985 and 1986. Her symptoms included burning on urination, vaginal discharge, cough, sharpness of breath, sore throat, severe abdominal pain, pelvic pain, convulsions and a severe drug reaction. In addition, Jamie was lethargic and depressed. What's more, on several occasions she said, "Mom, I'd rather be dead."

In September 1986 I called the International Health Foundation and was referred to a doctor in Dayton. He diagnosed a candida-related health problem and put Jamie on a comprehensive treatment program. It changed Jamie's life and the health of my family.

Today, May 1987, Jamie's a happy, healthy child. She hasn't been sick since last October. Her symptoms have all disappeared. Because of her terrible problems and her almost miraculous response to antiyeast treatment, I've organized a candida support group in Cincinnati. I want to spread the word so that others won't have to suffer like my little girl did.

At the age of 19 Jamie began to develop abdominal pain. A series of medical examinations showed she had endometriosis and when she called me I gave her the name of the late Dr. Arnold Kresch, a Palo Alto, California, board-certified gynecological surgeon who believed in the "yeast connection." Here are excerpts from my June 2001 phone visit with Jamie.

Dr. Kresch removed scar tissue adhesions and lasered off a lot of the endometriosis. He also took out the tumor and pretty much things have been good since then. Like with the stomach pains, every once in a while I'll get them, but they always said chances of me having kids was probably something that would never happen because of all the problems I'd had and because of the scar tissue that keeps coming back. I'm four months pregnant now. The doctors are shocked. Except for the problem with my gall bladder several weeks ago, I've been doing really good."

•• ••• •• ☒ •• ••• ••

I've kept up with Jamie and her mother over the years. I was thrilled when Jamie and her mother came to the International Health Foundation conferences in Dallas in 1987 and Memphis in 1988. They wanted to share Jamie's story with others.

We've exchanged letters and had conversations over the years and Jamie's mother, Sandy, gave me many favorable reports about Jamie and her progress through high school and on into college.

Dr. Crook

Paula

This 33-year-old woman gave a history of an active personal and professional life—very active. She worked ten hours a day, ran 15 miles a week, developed pimples and was put on tetracycline which she took for 18 months (between the ages of 27 and 29). After taking this antibiotic for several months, she began to develop concentration problems, anxiety, fatigue, depression and other symptoms.

She saw a number of physicians who said, "your problems are caused by stress." Yet, Paula's symptoms were so disabling that she had to give up her job and she stayed in bed most of every day.

Then, she found a physician who put her on nystatin, a sugar-free diet and nutritional supplements. Here are excerpts from a recent letter she sent me.

Thank you so much for writing your book. And thank the International Health Foundation for putting me in touch with the doctor who helped me. Rather than feeling like a limp wash cloth, I'm now back to 95% of where I started from. I have 10 to 14 hours of energy each day, although I do still get tired in the late afternoon and evening.

I'm writing you first to give you a progress report and next to send a small check with this letter for you to turn over to the International Health Foundation. I strongly believe in your efforts, so you can count me as an annual contributor.

Next, I want to tell you that I have been appalled, even embittered, by the lack of knowledge and resistance of doctors in this university medical center community about the relationship of superficial yeast infections to chronic illness. I realize that doctors and scientists are taught to believe in reliable information gathered in controlled studies and I suspect that malpractice litigation has strengthened that tendency.

But common sense should prevail when you and other doctors have gathered volumes of information that has returned so many chronic sufferers back to normal lives. It is truly beyond my comprehension why this information is so submerged. I would like to help raise the level of awareness, understanding and acceptance in this city. I go to church with the university's associate director for patient care services. I plan to meet with her and explore the reasons why there is such a deficit of acceptance and what would be needed to correct it.

I think that a good place to start would be with the nurses and physician assistants who work with health insurance companies. It would be in the best interest of the company to embrace this therapy because it is less expensive in both the short run, and in the long run. I also thought of these allied health workers for another reason. It would help them make their case before congressional committees on how their skills could be used to heal patients and reduce overall health care costs.

In my opinion, most traditional doctors are close-minded

due to the way they've been educated and also due to the horribly litiginous environment in America.

In the spring of 2001, Paula said, "I'm doing well. A supplement which I've found is very helpful is barley grass."

❀ ❀❀ ✉ ❀❀ ❀

Paula has been a friend of mine since the early 90s. We've talked on the phone many times and she's told me some of the things she's taken which have helped her. Included was barley grass! Like most people with candida-related problems, Paula has had a few ups and downs.

She also introduced me at a conference of businesswomen in Nashville several years ago and told everyone there her story. She serves as a member of the Advisory Board of the International Health Foundation.

Dr. Crook

Polly

May 2000

Dear Dr. Crook:

Thank you for your help in finding a physician in my area that is knowledgeable about yeast and its effect on the body. Below are the answers to the questions you inquired about in your letter sent about a month ago.

- I found a doctor in the Denver, CO area, about an hour and a half drive from Colorado Springs, that is in my HMO. Her name is Susanna Choi. Her office is located at 8200 E. Belleview Ave., Suite 240E, Greenwood Village, CO 80111.

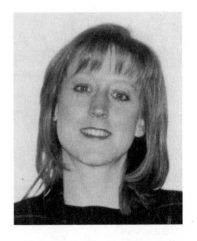

- I have been taking 200 mg of Diflucan for about 6 weeks with remarkable results. I will continue for 3 more weeks, then switch to nystatin. I also have been prescribed nystatin powder with the instruction to inhale to relieve nasal congestion and allergy symptoms.

⋄ My HMO, One Health, has covered the costs to date, including all 3 of my antifungal prescriptions.

⋄ My most troublesome symptoms were: fatigue, vaginal discharge, pain with intercourse, a multitude of digestive problems, more and stronger allergies, and lack of libido.

⋄ The 3 symptoms that bothered me the most were the fatigue, the digestive problems and the compounding allergies.

⋄ I am taking probiotics, a good vitamin/mineral supplement and magnesium potassium aspartate.

⋄ I have read *The Yeast Connection Handbook,* as well as many other holistic health titles, which speak to yeast overgrowth problems.

⋄ My partner has been very understanding. He feels that he probably has a yeast problem, but is too afraid of the diet to have it checked out. (He is a sugar-aholic.)

⋄ I believe my mother could have a yeast problem.

I feel that I have had great success so far with staying on a strict diet and taking Diflucan. My allergies have decreased significantly. My asthma has improved tremendously—I am now jogging! I no longer need 10 hours of sleep. And I have had no digestive system imbalance symptoms for quite some time.

I thank you from the bottom of my heart for your outstanding, pioneering work. If I can be of any further assistance, please let me know.

June 2000

I'm quite excited to report I keep getting better! My doctor (Susanna Choi) has taken me off of Diflucan after only 9 weeks. She is overjoyed by my progress. I am now taking nystatin, 4 times a day, and continuing on my diet. Though, I am allowed to cheat a bit.

I can't say that I have cheated much, however. I am feeling so incredible. I don't want to take any chances. The diet is a piece of cake, so to speak, once you've been on it for a few weeks. If you honor yourself and stick to it very stringently, the rewards far outweigh the things you give up. And it keeps getting easier. It is really nothing at all for me to ignore so many of the awful foods I used to love.

Regarding my previous letter, by all means, yes, you may use it in your next book. Whatever you feel will help get the message out to others feeling the same way I did. You have my permission to use all of my correspondence as you see fit.

In your first letter you asked me to speak about my asthma. I have been fortunate in that I did not start having asthma symptoms until about 10 years ago, when I was in my late 20s. I remember, even then, my allergies seemed to be getting out of control. For instance, I stopped reading the newspaper. It would make me sneeze uncontrollably. This was very frustrating since I never had any allergies growing up.

I know my diet wasn't as good as it used to be; I was on birth control for the umpteenth year; and I lived and breathed stress. I couldn't find enough energy to help myself out of that hole until I started wheezing from seemingly unnoticeable smells. This scared me. I went to see a doctor immediately and was told it wasn't a big deal, just "allergenic" asthma. Never mind that I had been very athletic growing up, even receiving an athletic scholarship for college.

I started reading about asthma. Most of the mainstream books say, "Once you get it, you'll have it for life. Here's how to deal with it." I became very depressed. I quit my job and started looking for a less stressful way to live my life. I did construction/renovation for a while to pay the bills. I enjoyed the work well enough until I contracted a serious case of bronchitis.

We were cleaning a filthy tin ceiling with a strong ammonia solution. Between the dirt and grime dropping down from above and the solution, my lungs were overwhelmed. I was down hard for over a week. Needless to say, my "allergenic" asthma got a significant boost. It took less to make me wheeze. It took almost nothing to make my eyes water and my nose sneeze. I began eating foods I knew were unhealthy as if I had no choice.

The wheezing frightened me so I stopped exercising. Eventually I cut way back on calories so I wouldn't gain too much from the lack of exercise even though I knew I was sacrificing much needed vitamins and minerals. I had recurring bouts of bronchitis off and on for four or five years, as I got weaker and weaker. It seemed to me moving out of Chicago and the city's smog might help. I moved to Colorado Springs in July of 1997.

I picked up a copy of one of you books on yeast-related health problems at a local health food store. It read like I was reading my own life story. I tried, unsuccessfully, to go on the diet giving up after a few days. Yet the similarities between the symptoms in your book and the way I constantly felt, haunted me. Finally I decided to follow your suggestion and see a doctor about the antifungal medications available that could help me in conjunction with the diet. I wrote to your nonprofit organization for help, finding a wonderful doctor from the list you sent me. There really isn't much to tell after that.

Just a Short Sweet Simple Recovery and My Life Back!

I am jogging—Colorado Springs is at 6000+ feet above sea level.

I hiked up to 10,500 feet last weekend and jogged back down.

I can read the newspaper without sneezing.

I can go down into my basement and look at old moldy comic books.

I have tons of energy with only 7 to 8 hours of sleep instead of the previously required 10+. The list goes on and on. It's as if the last 10 years of my life never existed. I realize you have heard this so many times before. Yet I can't help but say it again.

Thank you Dr. Crook!

Your work has completely changed my life.

⚬⚬⚬ ✉ ⚬⚬⚬

I had dinner with Polly and Mike in Colorado Springs in March 2001. She looked great and she told me she felt great.

Dr. Crook

Shannon

T wenty-six-year-old Shannon and her mother came in to see me in consultation on February 10, 1999, with complaints which affected every part of her body. Shannon's mother said,

When she was an infant she was troubled by colic for the first three months. Her formula was changed several times and she was finally put on nystatin. I can remember taking her to the doctor's office four times for colds and ear infections. During her toddler years she was troubled by many urinary tract infections. During grammar school, high school and her teen years she had continuous sinus and other respiratory infections. We kept Triaminic syrup in the house.

She also had more urinary problems in her teen years and took antibiotics many times. When she was about 18, I took her to urologist Lane Bicknell who carried out various procedures, including dilation of the urethra. She then took anti-infective medicines every day for two years—mainly Septra—but she also took a lot of other drugs. I'll let Shannon tell you more about her history.

Shannon said,

During my late teen years I was bothered by lots and lots of vaginal yeast infections. In an effort to control them, I used all sorts of vaginal creams.

My first child was born when I was 22, my second child at 24 and my third child at 26. After the birth of my third child on November 5, 1998, I began having severe migraine headaches. Since that time I've had all sorts of problems. I've seen many, many physicians and taken 25 prescription drugs. I've been hospitalized twice and stayed there for five days.

At times my pain and headaches were so severe the doctors gave me Demerol and Phenergan shots. Also, intravenous antibiotics. In an effort to find out what was causing my headaches, I was given two spinal taps and lots of other tests.

Through serendipity, I learned from Dr. Don Wilson's wife, Elizabeth, about yeast-related problems. I called and asked if I could see you and you said you had retired from practice and only saw a rare patient in consultation. You said you would only see me if my personal physician would refer me to you. By the time I got to see you, I was taking several other medicines in the doctor's efforts to help me. These included Amitriptyline (25 mg) and Xanax (0.25 mg) every night. I was also taking prenatal vitamins, primadophilus, ascorbic acid (1 tsp daily) and a product called Ultimate Fiber.

During your long discussion with me and my mother, you told me that anti-yeast treatment wouldn't be a quick fix for my problems. Yet you said that in your opinion, based on my history, you felt a therapeutic trial of a sugar-free diet and oral antiyeast medication was indicated. You told me to follow the diet instructions outlined in your book, *The Yeast*

Connection Handbook (pages 101–118 and 150–160) and to keep a daily diary of my symptoms.

Because my problems were so severe you recommended Diflucan, 200 mg once a day, until I showed significant improvement. And you told me I'd probably need to take it for one or two weeks—or even longer. Then you said that the dose might be reduced to 100 mg a day, but you said that every person was different.

You told me to continue the Primadophilus, 1 capsule three times a day and the nutritional supplements I was taking. You also told me to continue the Co-Enzyme Q_{10} which I had been taking three times a day and to discontinue the Ultimate Fiber and ascorbic acid.

After this visit I talked to you on the phone several times. I think it must have been four or five times. I told you I was following the diet faithfully and I felt a little better in some ways—less fatigue and not as much tingling. I was still bothered with lots of other symptoms, including urinary frequency and diarrhea.

Because of my symptoms, I was again seen by my neurologist who felt that further neurological investigation should be carried out, including an MRI. Then my vaginal and urinary symptoms were bothering me so much I went to Convenient Care where they told me my urine specimen was negative and gave me some vaginal creams.

On February 21st, you suggested I get my prescription for nystatin filled and take it three times a day, along with the Diflucan. When I called you on February 28th I told you that I felt very fatigued and continued to have other symptoms, including diarrhea, and I wondered if some of my symptoms could be caused by a die-off reaction from nystatin. You told me that you weren't certain but based on what I told you, because of the tendency of nystatin to cause die-off reactions, you suggested I stop the nystatin and resume the 200 mg daily dose of Diflucan until I was definitely better, then I might be able to cut it down.

You also told me it was okay to refill the Elavil prescription prescribed by my neurologist since it helped me rest and provided some relief from my numbness and tingling. In spite of your interest and care, I kept on having discouraging symptoms, although I was taking Diflucan, 200 mg a day, and following your diet. I had been eating some fruit and orange juice.

Some of my most troublesome symptoms were a feeling of pins and needles in my face, hands and back. Although I had had them for some time, they seemed to be getting worse. You told me to tighten up on my diet, leave off the fruits and juices, but to make sure that I took in enough calories so that I would maintain my nutrition, including fish, pork chops and other meats, and lots of vegetables.

You also recommended Atarax in a very small dose to see if it would help my symptoms and to see if I tolerated it. Because I'd had a bad reaction to an IV that contained Benadryl, Compazine and Toradol, I was concerned about a possible reaction to any medicine that was kin to Benadryl. You told me that in your experience Atarax was a very safe medicine and that the reaction I had from the IV probably wasn't due to Benadryl. You suggested that with the severity of my skin discomfort I should take the Atarax, beginning with ½ tsp and gradually building up to 2–3 tsp every four hours, if I tolerated it.

You also said that if my symptoms persisted or worsened, you might recommend discontinuing the Diflucan and shifting over to Lamisil. That's when you referred me to Dr. Paul Schwartz, the only general physician in Jackson who was a true believer in the yeast connection.

✦✦✦ ✉ ✦✦✦

In the late winter of 2001 I walked in the office of a small company in Jackson. The receptionist wasn't at her desk so I took a few steps down the hall when a beautiful young lady walked up and gave me a hug. She said, "I'm Shannon. Thank you, thank you, thank you. You and Dr. Schwartz saved my life."

Shannon's story is typical in so many, many ways. Antibiotics were given to her on many occasions during her infancy, childhood and teen years; visits to many fine physicians and specialists who were doing their best to help her. Although she took medications of all kinds—nothing seemed to help. Her battle to get her yeast under control wasn't easy—it rarely is—and required courage, patience and persistence.

Dr. Crook

Virginia

ecause of acne, this teenager was put on tetracycline early in 1991. A short time later, Virginia said,

I became extremely tired. I ached all over and developed severe headaches. In the 18 months since that time, I've been tired, weak and depressed.

Virginia saw a number of physicians and several medications were tried, including antidepressant. Because of her persistent symptoms, she was unable to go to school and the school provided a homebound teacher. Weakness and daily severe headache were her worst symptoms.

I saw Virginia the first time in September 1992. And at the conclusion of my office history, I made the following diagnostic impression:

"Chronic Fatigue Syndrome triggered by a combination of circumstances. My first bet would be yeast overgrowth triggered by broad-spectrum antibiotics. There may be secondary nutritional deficiencies, food sensitivities and reactivation of latent viruses."

I recommended a sugar-free, dairy-free special diet, preparations of Lactobacillus acidophilus, and nutritional supplements. After 10 days I prescribed Diflucan, 200 mgs a day for three days, then 100 mgs. a day.

Virginia improved steadily and by Thanksgiving she was able

to return to school. And in a letter I sent to Virginia and her mother on December 7, 1992, I said:

Dear Friends. I'm delighted at Virginia's improvement and I commend you both for following the treatment program. I feel the diet, Diflucan and nutritional supplements made a difference . . . Even though some of your doctors may be skeptical!

Virginia, I look upon you as a normal, healthy young woman. Continue to eat a good diet and don't cheat too often. Cut your dose of Diflucan to every other day, then if you do well, discontinue it after Christmas.

You can walk and carry on your usual activities, but do not exercise vigorously—such as running or jogging long distances—for at least three months. If you're having problems of any type which relate to your previous illness, and you feel I could help, please call.

I called Virginia in January 1994 to get a follow-up report. She told me she was doing great and that she hadn't missed any school. No headache, no fatigue. When I asked her about her diet and medication, she said:

Of course, I cheat on my diet at times, but I still consume a much better diet than most teenagers. I take the vitamins you prescribed, Kyolic odor-free garlic and a preparation of *Lactobacillus acidophilus.*

In the spring of 1994, Virginia ran into problems. She developed a urinary tract infection and was put on antibiotics. A short time later, many of her symptoms returned. What's more she developed mental confusion and other symptoms which landed her in the emergency room. Then, and I'm not sure how or why it happened, they put her in a mental hospital for about a week before she was able to get out.

I renewed her prescription for Diflucan and told her to tighten up on her diet. Yet, because she continued to be depressed, her family physician gave her Prozac to take along with the Diflucan. Again she improved.

After three weeks, Virginia was able to taper off the Prozac and then stop it, and she remained symptom free. Then, in another two weeks, nystatin was substituted for the Diflucan. Here's another therapeutic intervention which helped her: a thyroid supplement. Because Virginia's morning oral temperature readings were low (96.8–97.4 degrees), I prescribed 32 mg. of USP thyroid once a day, in addition to other treatment measures.

In September 1994, I spoke to Virginia's mother, who said:

Virginia is doing great. She's back in school and doing well and has an after school hours job.

In November 1994, Virginia's mother called. Here's a report.

Virginia is a healthy, happy young woman. She's a senior in high school and has recently been selected to represent her class in a course which will be held in Jackson. She continues to follow her diet—most of the time—and she takes her nutritional supplements and nystatin and acidophilus once a day. I really feel like she's out of the woods.

✧✧✧ ✉ ✧✧✧

I haven't talked to Virginia in several years, but from reports I've received from friends and relatives, she graduated from the University of Tennessee in Knoxville and is now taking care of her two young children.

Dr. Crook

Women in Their 40s and 50s

Anita

This major in the U.S. Marine Corps wrote me a long letter in 1992. She told me that she had been troubled with yeast-related chronic fatigue syndrome for several years. Although she improved on a comprehensive treatment program which included nystatin, nutritional supplements and other therapies, she was still experiencing problems.

In responding, I sent her a packet of information including comments about Diflucan. She took this information to her physician and obtained a prescription for this new antifungal medication. She also tightened up on her diet.

A few weeks later, during a trip to California, I met Anita and she told me she had improved significantly. As I gathered material for this book, I asked her to give me a summary of her story. Here it is:

I was the "typical" CFS profile: Female; 30s; educated; a workaholic. I hold two law degrees and was a Major in the U.S. Marine Corps. I never took sick leave, and I often took antibiotics for a chronic urinary tract infection.

In January 1985 1 became desperately ill. I slept 14 hours a day, my head felt as though it would burst, I ached all over, especially my joints. Just getting dressed exhausted me.

My allergies were so bad I took up to 15 antihistamines a day. Doctors could find nothing wrong. First there was concern from the naval establishment, then nonchalance, then disdain. I considered suicide. I didn't know how I would ever be able to perform my job, but I had to work to support myself.

I began reading everything I could find on diseases with my symptomatology and in March 1987 I ran across an article written by Arthur Kaslow, M.D., in *Let's Live Magazine* discussing Epstein-Barr/CFS. I made an appointment with Dr. Kaslow, who offered not only superb medical care, but concern and compassion as well.

He started me on nystatin, daily injections of B$_{12}$, plus other nutrients. I changed my diet to one of whole foods, supplemental vitamins and minerals. I added acidophilus and a colon cleanser. Changes did not occur overnight, but I slowly turned the corner back toward the living.

Dr. Kaslow passed away some time ago, leaving those of us whose lives he changed with a great void. He was a fine man who made a positive contribution to others. He is sorely missed.

I have continued to read and study about CFS and yeast infections and this year I had all my mercury amalgams removed. I've modified my diet over the last few years so I eat mostly organically grown whole grains and vegetables, limited fruit and a small amount of fish, fowl and meat.

Do I eat this well consistently? No. I still crave sweets and still adore coffee. I try to do the best I can under all circumstances and not worry too much. One thing is certain. In my case, there's no hope of ever controlling CFS unless the underlying yeast condition is treated . . .

I am in control again, but all my priorities have changed.

I no longer sleep in the office because I have so much work to do. I have a good laugh every day.

Anita resigned her commission, which she had held with the Marine Corps for thirteen years and opened a private practice in Texas in 1994. Today, 2001, Anita has ten lawyers working under her supervision and enjoys excellent health. She also lives in the country and, for recreation, she rides the horses she's always loved. In a recent conversation, she said she would be delighted to share her story with others as she wants to help other people with CFS.

➳➳➳ ✉ ➳➳➳

I first met Anita in California in the early 90s and she appeared with me on the taping of a program for a national TV network. Then, according to information I received, the show changed producers and the program was never aired.

Dr. Crook

Beverly

D ear Dr. Crook,

I am happy to share my story with you and your readers. Around the age of 40, I began to have vague symptoms—dizziness, exhaustion, joint pain (especially upon arising), abdominal bloating and cravings for sweets. I also felt as though I had a box covering my head and could only see out the eye-holes. Since I had trouble with irregular menses, my GYN put me on birth control pills. They helped the periods to normalize but my blood pressure started to rise so high I was placed on anti-hypertensives.

Then came a weird symptom. I had dizziness whenever I lay my head down at night. For this, I was placed on Meclizine. My primary M.D. thought I was suffering from depression and wanted to give me yet another medication. As a once healthy person, I felt as though I was falling apart all at once! Taking medication was not something I wanted to do for the rest of my life so I took it upon myself to seek out the opinion of an alternative medicine physician. I had heard of Dr. Ray Wunderlich Jr., M.D., in St. Petersburg, FL.

So in May of 2000, I had my first encounter with him. He took one look at me and said, "you look as though you have candida." I had no idea what that was but took his suggestions for successful treatment. He recommended the anti-stress diet which is similar to the cave man diet: no sweets (even fruits), yeast, dairy, grains or breads for the first 6 weeks along with taking Ultra-Flora DF 2 in the A.M. and P.M.

Being a vegetarian most of my life, I must say it took some willpower to remain on this diet. Most of my meals consisted of salads, cooked, raw, and steamed veggies and lots of nuts, seeds and their butters. But after a week, the sugar cravings disappeared and the weight started to drop. It has been over a year now and I have lost 40 pounds. I continue to remain on this diet but occasionally eat pasta, rice and one piece of fruit per week.

Needless to say, I am no longer on any prescription medication and my "old age symptoms have disappeared. I owe it all to the man who diagnosed me correctly and helped me realize what an important factor diet plays in our well-being. I was so pleased with my successful treatment that I now work for Dr. Wunderlich as one of his staff R.N.s. It's amazing how many people are treated with prescription medication for their symptoms rather than looking for the cause.

Thank you for the opportunity to share this with your readers. I hope this will help open their eyes and encourage them to take their health problems in their own hands.

Sincerely,
Beverly Curry

⚬⚬⚬ ✉ ⚬⚬⚬

I've known Ray Wunderlich for 25 years. Like me, he was trained as a pediatrician. For 20 years, he's been interested in helping people with yeast-related health problems. His comments which I included in my 1986 book, **The Yeast Connection** can be found in Section VI of this book.

Dr. Crook

Carol

Life is full of ironies, isn't it! While growing up on a farm in eastern Nebraska, wheat supported us and paid for my college tuition. I married into a wheat-farming family and began my ritual of making delicious, homemade bread. After all, I had to support the family business, didn't I!

But, since my teens, recurring sinus infections required frequent, prolonged doses of antibiotics—sometimes a year at a time—and worsened as I grew older. Ironically, I eventually learned that avoiding wheat eliminated the sinus infections, but I still didn't feel well.

I suspected candida as the reason, but I couldn't find anyone who would talk to me about it. In fact, I remember lying on an examining table, with a nurse whispering in my ear, "You're full of candida". Yet no official diagnosis appeared on my medical chart and her secretive demeanor puzzled me.

And now comes the fortuitous part. I was doing a book signing at a local health food store where Kathy Gibbons, Ph.D., a biochemist/nutritionist told me of her work and Dr. Crook's writings. Working with Dr. Gibbons, and the gynecologist she then worked with, Dr. Susanna Choi, I began the road to recovery with Diflucan and a yeast-free diet as my allies.

Today, I maintain a constant rotation of anti-fungals recommended in Dr. Crook's books and an occasional month of Diflucan when circumstances, such as surgery, require antibiotics. I know the yeast-free lifestyle is just that—a way of life that I will follow forever.

Carol Fenster, Ph.D.

✉

Carol is the author of **Special Diet Solutions: Healthy Cooking Without Wheat, Gluten, Dairy, Eggs, Yeast, or Refined Sugar.** *This book is available at Savory Palate Press, PMB #404, 8174 South Holly, Littleton, CO 80122–4004*

I had lunch with Carol in Denver in May 2001. She's about the same age as my daughters and, like them, she's a beautiful lady.

Dr. Crook

Elizabeth

Dear Dr. Crook:

Thank you for your efforts to educate doctors and patients throughout the world on the many health problems related to Candida Related Complex (CRC). CRC has impacted my health since the day I was born. I was a very sickly child for the first twenty-one years of my life due to a combination of improper feeding and frequent antibiotics. During the 1950s it was popular to use infant baby formula and start feeding infants solid foods at two weeks of age. This combination caused severe distress to my immune system and I suffered from severe hay fever and several bouts of sore throats, ear infections, pneumonia, and coughs. My tonsils were removed at age seven but this did nothing to alleviate my condition.

The damage from the multiple courses of antibiotics to my intestinal environment caused severe constipation and acne during my teens years. This resulted in even more drug therapies that aggravated my CRC—the antibiotic tetracycline for two years and birth control pills.

At the age of twenty-two I finally became exposed to information about diet, nutrition and natural healing. A chiropractor taught me that susceptibility to infections was not so much caused by the strength of the germ as the weakness of our immune system. He taught me that consuming a diet rich in simple sugars and flour products was like throwing a party for bad germs. If you stop feeding the germs they will stop growing out of control. In the twenty-six years since that time, I have never again used antibiotics to treat an infection and my hay fever is totally gone. The same information that prevents bacterial infections also helped me get my yeast imbalances under control. Over the years I have used nystatin and some natural antifungals but they were never effective for very long unless I stayed on track with a diet rich in whole foods and devoid of junk. My body has felt like the "canary in the coal mine" but I now realize that those foods, etc. that I am sensitive to are very destructive to my health.

In 1980, I started developing an autoimmune disorder caused by several toxic exposures such as formaldehyde, mercury and some heat-damaged allergy shots. My illness included multiple, daily hive attacks, severe insomnia, fatigue, multiple chemical sensitivities, severe bloating and gas, menstrual problems and heavy bleeding, nosebleeds, brain fog, and thyroid and adrenal problems. Improving my diet, digestion, elimination and intestinal health has been the key to reversing my symptoms and getting well.

Even though I initially cursed my health problems, my road to recovery has enabled me to become a much better physician with a unique perspective on how to figure out some of the complex problems that come about when the integrity of the intestinal tract is damaged. It is very gratifying to patients who regain control of their lives and health when yeast and other bad germs are brought under control with a healthy diet and the proper nutritional supplements and medications.

Elizabeth Walker, D.C.

Author of *Conquer Fatigue in 30 Days*

Jackie

In 1992, I was a patient at the National Jewish Hospital in Denver, Colorado, and with their help, I was able to continue working as a School Office Manager in the Cherry Creek Schools. For exercise, I would walk around a short block, stopping several times to catch my breath, to administer medication, or to get my heart rate down. My husband would go with me because he wasn't sure that I would make it back home without assistance.

My problems were not obesity, but chronic sinusitis (from my teenage years) and asthma (from the early 80's). The sinus problems heightened the asthma problems, and the only way to combat this was to increase the strength of my medications which included Ventolin, Benconase AQ, Azmacort, Intal, Provera and numerous antibiotics.

I had sought help from various specialists, such as allergists; ear, nose and throat doctors; and neurologists. Two sinus surgeries in '81 and '90 had given me temporary relief which was certainly welcome at the time, but they were definitely not long-term solutions. (The only long-term effect was decreased sense of smell.)

I was 52 years old and felt considerably older. My headaches were frequent and often severe. The constant mucus draining in the back of my throat was thick green and yellow with red blood spots which gave me a perpetual sore throat and often affected my speech.

My primary physician was concerned because I was taking antibiotics every three or four months and becoming allergic to everything he tried which is why he finally sent me to National Jewish Hospital. It was necessary to keep Benadryl handy to treat allergic reactions to foods and medications. As a result, I couldn't clean our home because of my allergic reaction to dust. I couldn't sit next to someone wearing perfume or where there might be smokers present.

I was constantly fatigued, sleeping 12 to 16 hours, and never getting enough rest. I was frightened when I'd wake up with numb hands, arms, and/or legs. There were times after my work day when I would literally crawl upstairs to bed and pray for the weekends when I could sleep longer. I often blamed my fuzzy thinking, poor performance, and graying hair on just "getting older."

During this time I was extremely depressed. It wasn't a life worth living. My husband's brother, a physician, had advised my husband to be prepared for the worst possible outcome. One afternoon while observing patients pull their oxygen tanks to their appointments at National Jewish, I became angry. I realized that this was my destiny if I continued under the same program. I was determined to do something to change that outcome.

I told my physician that I wanted to read everything I could because I was going to find a way to get well. He agreed that I should read and become knowledgeable about asthma (I had attended numerous classes about how to live with asthma at National Jewish), but I could tell, from the look he exchanged with his nurse, he thought I was not being realistic or practical about changing my condition. They had informed me that the asthma generally gets progressively worse for their patients if you also suffer from sinus problems.

I started reading numerous books and articles and began following a diet recommended in a book about food allergies. A friend recommended that I read *Sinus Survival* by Dr. Ivker. I couldn't believe how much he knew "about me," and I was pleased to learn that he was in Colorado.

I talked with my husband about seeking Dr. Ivker's help, and he said, "What have you got to lose?" Dr. Ivker recommended that I continue with the diet, although he predicted I would have numerous allergies.

At the end of my test diet, I tested out allergic to everything I ate, except soy. I was equally surprised to hear Dr. Ivker say that he could take me off all my medications and cure my sinus and asthma problems. It was almost too good to be true, and I wondered how this could be possible when so many physicians had told me the opposite.

Dr. Ivker placed me on the physical aspect of the program first with environmental changes and vitamins and herbs which gave me immediate, positive improvement. However, I found it necessary to complete the total program (physical, mental, social, spiritual, and emotional) to gain total freedom from my past illnesses.

Under Dr. Ivker's care, my skin lost its gray hue, my hair stopped graying, and I regained my health. Much that I had attributed to "old age" was actually just poor physical health. The goal was to improve my respiratory and immune systems so that my body could care for and protect itself. This was accomplished to the degree that in 1994, I participated in "Ride the Rockies," a 413-mile bike tour through the Colorado Rocky Mountains. Since then I have ridden in three more "Ride the Rockies" tours with family and friends.

As a result of Dr. Ivker's program I have a life again. When I started the Sinus Survival program, I was about a 2–3 on a scale of 1 to 10. Today I am in the 8–10 range.

I took Nizoral and Flora Balance for the yeast problem, along with the vitamins and herbs under Dr. Ivker's care. He was also treating me for asthma and chronic sinus problems which he said were the result of a very weakened respiratory and immune system, and the very first item on his list was to treat the yeast problem.

I still work on my diet and do my exercises and my husband and I are making plans for our retirement. This will include traveling, reading, riding our bikes, visiting our children, and enjoying this beautiful world. As Dr. Ivker predicted, I no longer need to take medications for sinusitis, asthma or any other illnesses.

Sinus Survival is not a "quick fix," it takes commitment, dedication, time, and communication. Searching and preparing a variety of foods different from our "normal" menu, accepting that I had anger, realizing that this is a life change (not just for a day, week, or month), all required blind faith in Dr. Ivker's vast accumulation of knowledge and experience.

If you are starting this program, you may struggle and wonder "Why bother, it's not worth it?" Try to remember that "you are doing the best you can" and that this program is about nourishing the entire being, the mind, the body, and the spirit. Let me assure you that it is worth the effort. The sinus survival program gives you the tools you need to rebuild your body and mind and soul, which in turn gives you good health, joy, and happiness as you take control of your own life.

❖ ❖❖ ✉ ❖❖ ❖

Dr. Bob Ivker lives in Colorado and I was thrilled to read the first edition of his book **Sinus Survival.** *He also is a recent president of the American Holistic Medical Association. His book is now a bestseller and can be found in all health food stores and bookstores.*

Dr. Crook

Jeanette*

I n 1982, Jeanette, a physician's daughter, came to see me searching for help. Here are excerpts from a letter she sent me prior to our first visit.

I'm ready to find out if it's "all in my head" and my symptoms are due to "just getting older" or whether there's something that's really making me sick.

Jeanette then told me about many of the symptoms which had bothered her for years, including abdominal pain, aching in her fingers, headache, dizziness, nausea, persistent night cough, chest pain and chemical sensitivities, and she said:

This spring I developed bladder problems; two infections and frequent urination. I've also been unable to empty my bladder without hard pushing. These symptoms took me to a urologist who diagnosed it as "a small urethra and spasm."

He dilated me and gave medicine. Incidentally, frequent urination had been a part of my life, but not the pressure. (I have even wet the bed since I've been married.) I also am bothered by nervousness, fatigue, puffiness in my fingers, bloating, excessive weight gain and breast soreness during the week before my period.

---

*Not her real name.

On a simple but comprehensive treatment program which featured nystatin, dietary changes and nutritional supplements, Jeanette steadily improved. She moved to an adjoining state in 1985 and although I haven't seen her as a patient since that time, I've kept in touch with her through occasional letters and phone calls. And I knew she was doing well. To get an update I wrote her in March 1993 and asked her to send me a progress report. Here are excerpts from her letter:

Thanks for your letter. I'm doing quite well and enjoying my forties healthwise much more than my thirties. I'm 43 now and am quite busy with three children. One almost 17, one 14 and one 5. I operate with my energy level much higher today than when we first began the 'yeast journey' together.

I still don't eat bread, but I do have yeast in my diet, some sugar and other junk. But overall my eating is much healthier than ten years ago.

⚫⚫⚫ ✉ ⚫⚫⚫

I haven't talked to Jeanette in the past several years and I hope she's continuing to do well.

Dr. Crook

Joyce

n August 1992, this 33-year-old woman called me on the IHF Hotline. She said:

I've had severe myasthenia gravis (MG) for over 20 years and have been troubled by many other symptoms. I recently obtained a copy of your book, *The Yeast Connection*, and began to change my diet. I'm already improving! I'm off all MG medication and gaining back my strength.

Joyce also told me she had taken many antibiotics during infancy and early childhood, and that she had been troubled by recurrent vaginal yeast infections in childhood and early adolescence. At the age of 13 she began to show symptoms which led to the diagnosis of MG. Her symptoms at that time included: completely nasal voice—air came out of her nose instead of her mouth when she spoke; she was unable to swallow and had to wash down food with liquid. Joyce had no control of muscles in her face. She was unable to smile and her eyes remained open when sleeping— she was uncoordinated and troubled by double vision, migraine headaches, and stomachaches.

In subsequent letters, Joyce sent me further details about her illness. She said:

I was tired all the time and slept a lot and was unable to wake up in the morning for school. I was also troubled by sinus drainage and mucus. At the time I was diagnosed at 13, I had only 20% of my body strength left and weighed only 89 lbs.

During the years following the diagnosis, many therapies were tried, including removal of my thymus gland three weeks after diagnosis; prednisone, 100 mgs. on alternate days for 14 years.

Then at the age of 21, following another positive blood test for MG, I was placed on Mestinon and a year later I began taking Mytelase. Between ages 21 and 32, my symptoms of MG improved, yet I was troubled by recurring yeast infections, constipation, depression, recurrent colds and flu, some eyelid weakness and insomnia. I was a chocoholic and sugarholic craving these things almost constantly.

In 1990, at the age of 32, the MG became full blown again, this time with severe body weakness. I took additional medications, including daily prednisone and gamma globulin by intravenous drip, once a week. Also the dose of Mytelase was increased from 20 mgs. to 46 mgs. daily.

In spite of these therapies, in 1992 Joyce continued to be troubled by many symptoms, including PMS, headache, irritability, panic attacks, poor memory and "indescribable" body weakness and fatigue, insomnia and depression.

I had to be vertical most of the day. I could not carry on normal duties, including cooking and cleaning. I had to quit my job. Some days I had to stay in bed all day—folding a load of clothes required too much energy.

My right eye drooped in various degrees and the right

corner of my mouth felt numb or weak. My right eye remained open at night causing extreme pain.

After reading your book and talking to you in August 1992, I began a sugar-free, yeast-free diet. I also eliminated all fruits, white rice, white pasta, white flour, and all refined processed foods and dairy products, with the exception of real butter, yeast products, fermented products, manmade fats and oils. Any of the above foods would bring back my symptoms, especially the sweets, which caused weak days to return.

Within a week or so the constipation and fatigue began improving and I had more good days than bad days. In addition, my memory began to improve, so did the PMS and depression. The panic/anxiety attacks disappeared completely. However, my right eye continued to droop, which never really improved on the MG medications; so did the right corner of my mouth and I was still bothered by my right eye staying open at night.

Because of Joyce's history of recurrent yeast infections, improvement following dietary changes and Dr. Truss' success in treating patients with MG using nystatin and diet, I wrote to her and said, "Call or write Dr. Truss. I feel he may be able to help you."

Early in 1993, Joyce went to Birmingham to see Dr. Truss. Following a careful history and examination, he prescribed nystatin, ½ tsp. four times a day, along with vaginal nystatin twice daily. He also stressed the importance of carefully following a restricted diet and suggested she limit carbohydrates to 80 mg per day, which she did.

Within a short time, she reported greater improvement, including 100% more energy; no more "weak" days. She said, however,

I had symptoms if I ate any of the foods I had been avoiding—especially fruits and healthy sweets, those sweetened with brown rice syrup.

In March 1993, I went on a ski vacation and skied from 7:30 in the morning to 4:30 in the evening! By contrast, seven months earlier, I couldn't sit up or do other normal household duties. My memory showed remarkable improvement—100% better—especially with recall. The depression also improved 100%.

I actually felt happy. The PMS disappeared and so did the yeast infections. I still have some sinus drainage, but no more bronchitis or sinusitis.

I also noticed double vision which is present 100% of the time is improving and I am able to pull the two images together. Prior to the diet and nystatin I was unable to do this. I noticed a tremendous improvement in the weakness and numbness in the corner of my mouth and my right eye no longer stayed open at night. I no longer test positive for MG.

Symptoms that still bothered me included droopiness of the right eye, some irritability at times and cold hands and cold feet.

In the late summer of 1993 Joyce wrote and told me that she was continuing to do well, yet she was still troubled by weakness in her eyelids and right corner of her mouth. She also said that

₩₩ꩰ these symptoms still present, MG specialists would question the success of the diet, even though their method of treatment had also failed in controlling this symptom. She also said:

Prior to avoiding sugar and fruits and making other changes in my diet, I had constant problems with colds and flu. For example, I had almost a dozen spells of colds, flu, sinusitis, bronchitis in a 12 month period. Now, since being on the diet, I have recovered without antibiotics for the first time. And I've had only one flu attack in the 12 month period since starting the diet. That attack happened four days after drinking a glass of punch with sugar in it.

Then in a letter I received in October 1993, Joyce said that Dr. Truss had increased her dose of nystatin and that she now has days when her eyelids are completely balanced and she feels fine. And she said,

The treatment is working!! The only thing is—I absolutely have to get the oral and vaginal doses done as instructed. I ran out of nystatin and lost the improvement. Now I'm getting it back. I also have to do the vaginal dose. If I miss even one time, the improvement lessens.

I also tested fruit and lost the improvement. I also tested frozen Rice Dream (sweetened with brown rice syrup) and lost the improvement. The loss is only temporary, but confirms what is taking place.

Conclusion: Taking the proper dose of nystatin regularly, orally and vaginally, restricting carbohydrates, and staying away from all sweets, as well as junk food, white flour, white rice, and all refined foods is crucial to the recovery of a myasthenic. Sweets (even so-called "healthy sweets" like fruit, honey, rice syrup, maple syrup, etc.) are my number one enemy. I'm sure other MG victims will experience this also.

In your books you've mentioned the importance of a positive attitude and faith in God. God healed me by following the diets in your book and I will eat a healthy diet the rest of my life.

I continued to hear from Joyce over the next several years and in February 1998 she wrote me telling me of some of her ups and downs. Here are excerpts from her letter.

Initially, I did very well on the Vegan Diet and I even went further with a Vegan raw food diet which helped me overcome my problems with constipation. I also felt fine without the nystatin. I did well for about 18 months. Then in mid-1996, I surprisingly lost all improvement in my bowel movements that the Vegan Diet brought. I also began to have body weakness and difficulty sleeping, constipation, anxiety, heart racing and wind-like sounds in my ears. My health continued to get worse.

By March 1997, 1 decided to go back on the Lederle nystatin. My insurance now covered it. I also decided to go on a carbohydrate restricted diet as well and eat more animal protein. I met with Dr. Douglas Sandberg* at the University of Miami Medical School and he helped me get back on the

*Dr. Sandberg retired from his position as Professor of Pediatrics on January 15, 1998.

anti-candida program. I counted carbohydrates for about four months, not getting over a maximum of 80 grams a day.

I worked up to one teaspoon of nystatin oral powder, five times a day, before I got needed results, plus one capsule vaginally twice daily. I'm currently on the anti-candida diet, and I'm still watching closely my carbohydrate intake and I still take the same amount of nystatin. My improvement has continued, I have regained the ground I lost, and I fully expect to be symptom-free.

With Dr. Sandberg's help, I was able to determine what had gone wrong. The Vegan Diet fed the candida, since it involves eating large amounts of carbohydrates even though I ate healthy carbohydrates—whole grains, vegetables and legumes. Also, going off the nystatin was not good.

It has now been almost a year since I started back on the anti-candida program and I have regained the ground I lost, plus I am now getting rid of other symptoms. My elimination is very good and my right eyelid is getting better. Some days it does not sag at all! I would tell anyone with a yeast-related problem: 1) Don't go off the nystatin and 2) Don't go on a Vegan or vegetarian diet or any animal protein-free diet, especially where carbohydrates are high, because doing those two things set me back.

In August 2001, Joyce wrote me and said,

For quite a while I was taking 2 tsp. of nystatin powder five times a day and twice vaginally. I discontinued this when Lederle stopped making nystatin. Other brands of nystatin upset my stomach terribly. I did okay off the nystatin, which

I attributed to the diet, prayer and taking an excellent probiotic (friendly bacteria replacement), "Health Trinity."

Then after discussion with you, a maintenance dose of Diflucan seemed like a good idea. Although my energy level and health is excellent, you explained that a maintenance dose of an antifungal would help prevent a yeast overgrowth reoccurrence.

I continue the anti-candida diet strictly and will *forever!* My diet consists of organic beef, turkey and chicken, vegetables, nuts, seeds and whole grains. I take 200 mg of Diflucan twice a week. I am on my third week and doing very well, with lots of energy and no symptoms of candida or other illness. I did notice some die-off, thrush in my mouth and craving sweets at first.

I continue to telephone counsel many who want to go on the diet and have MG patients call me from all over the country. All have improved who follow your protocol.

The best test for my recovery is not in a hospital lab or doctor's office, but at home where I care for the needs of my family, including my husband who has a very demanding career; and perhaps the real test, our two-year-old and one-year-old sons.

I meet the challenges of each day with a smile of victory because I know I have won the battle against MG and candida yeast. I thank the Lord God for your diet and the help it is bringing so many.

✦✦✦ ✉ ✦✦✦

In July 2001 Joyce called and told me she was experiencing problems in obtaining nystatin that would agree with her so her physician prescribed Diflucan. Joyce's wonderful story shows clearly that people who are winning the battle against yeast are courageous, persistent and almost always experience ups and downs. Joyce and her husband came up from Miami to Orlando to have lunch with me several years ago. During the past several years, she's been writing and calling to help other people with myasthenia gravis and/or other chronic health problems.

Dr. Crook

Kay

I suffered for almost 10 years, 8 doctors, laparoscopic examinations, dilatation of the urethra, etc.

In 1989 I read Dr. Larrian Gillespie's book, *You Don't Have to Live With Cystitis*. With the help and encouragement of my husband, I saw Dr. Gillespie in February 1989. After a week of tests and surgery she confirmed that I did have a disease and it had a name, interstitial cystitis. On the downside—no cure.

After returning home I began Dr. Gillespie's IC diet immediately. I also had six treatments with DMSO, plus bicarbonate and steroids. *Gradually*, over the next year, I improved so much I was able to go water skiing, snow sledding and enjoy all sorts of everyday activities. I still had to follow my diet. I kept a food diary for two years to test foods that increased my pain.

Then in spite of various therapies, my troubles came back. By the second summer I was bright red in the vulva, had constant discharge and pelvic pain. Numerous trips to the gynecologist proved useless. And they'd say, "No yeast infection."

So I went to the health food store and ran into Jodi Taylor-Smith—a woman who had tried to help me before without too much success. She suggested an antiyeast program, including vitamins and garlic and a diet free of sugar and yeast. This time I experienced some improvement.

Then I went to Dr. Betty Raney in Zionsville, my new

gynecologist, who was very sympathetic to IC and yeast and started me on Diflucan, 100 mg. every other day. I have improved, but sometimes I still have vaginal itching and discharge (much milder, but still there), headache and fatigue, especially 3 or 4 days before my period.

I know I am not alone . . . there are thousands of women suffering some of the same problems or there wouldn't be nightly commercials for Gyne-Lotrimin and Monistat 7.

February 1994 Progress Report

I'm doing great—terrific. I would not even know most days that I ever had IC. It's absolutely incredible. I can sleep 6 or 7 hours and never get up.

Other symptoms which once bothered me, including eczema on my hand, cleared. And my sinus/allergy symptoms are almost non-existent.

As far as the frequency and the pain and the pressure and just feeling like your bladder's on fire, all of the symptoms that I had in '89 and before are all so much better. It's just unbelievable. I occasionally have some vaginal problems, yet when I do I know it's because I cheated with sugar and things like that.

I'm still taking the 100 mg. of Diflucan every other day, plus nutritional supplements, including dairy-free strains of the good bacteria *Lactobacillus acidophilus*.

February 1998 Progress Report

There's none of the burning, the urgency, the inability to hardly be able to start the urine flow. I go to bed about 10 and get up about 6 and I rarely have to get up during the night. I may go 4–5 times during the day—not anything out of the ordinary. In fact, there are times when I go all morning at teaching and forget to go to the bathroom.

If I have any symptoms, which are rare, it's usually a few days before my period. I'm experiencing a wonderful level of wellness and I want to learn more. I want to know more about what I can do for my family and myself just to stay well and be healthier.

I continue to see Dr. Raney and Meg Moorman, the wonderful nurse practitioner who works with her. And when I experienced a flare-up of IC symptoms (which has happened only twice in the past 4 years), they put me on Diflucan three years ago, 100 mgs. a day for 20–30 days. I feel like if I take any less than that, I'm not really getting things back under control. Diflucan really saved my life.

When I read those ads about 1–2 doses of Diflucan in a magazine, it upsets me. Maybe it's o.k. for a woman who has a simple yeast infection for the first time. If the woman is a chronic yeast patient and has IC-related symptoms, she'll have to take it much longer and be willing to work with the diet. I took Diflucan for almost six months the first time and it took me that long to get rid of my vulvodynia.

Today, I do a lot of other things, including diet, exercise, stress management and nutritional supplements, including a teaspoon of probiotics each day.

•••• ⊠ ••••

I've had dinner with Kay on two occasions and she and a friend appeared with Dr. Phillip Mosbaugh and me on TV in Indianapolis.
Dr. Crook

Linda

I was just really sick for a long time. I was really tired and everything. We happened to come home on leave—my husband was in the military. This was in the mid 1980s. My Mom had been telling her chiropractor how sick I was. He had a copy of *The Yeast Connection*. He gave it to my Mom to loan to me to read. So I took it home with me and read it. Not too long after that I wrote to you begging for help. You were so kind to write back and tell me about the yeast problem.

The Air Force sent me all over town and I saw at least a dozen different doctors and specialists. They couldn't find anything wrong. They did find a prolapsed mitral valve. You had given me a doctor's name in South Dakota—Dr. Argabright. He's retired now. He told me that it wasn't going to take a short time to get well. He was right about that. He was the first person to put me on nystatin.

I was so tired. I had a reflux problem with burning in my esophagus. The doctors kept telling me there was nothing wrong with me. I had two endoscopies over a year and a half. I was weak and tired and I ached all over. Then I saw Dr. Penn, an epidemiologist. He was very kind to me. I was also chemically sensitive and having a hard time going anywhere. I lost weight down to about 94 lbs. That's when I ended up in the hospital.

In fact, my daughter, Sally, even talked to Dr. Penn one

day when he was in my room. They talked about some sort of test they might do to look for the yeast, but they couldn't find anything. From there I went to the mental hospital for another two weeks. They took away everything, including my nystatin and my vitamins. It took me about a week to get those back.

I had taken your first book, *The Yeast Connection,* with me to the hospital. They told me I could have a heart attack at any time. So basically they turned me over to a psychiatrist when they couldn't find anything wrong with me. Then I went off my diet and I ate everything in sight just to gain weight because they told me I couldn't get out until I was over 100 lbs. It took me two and a half weeks to do that. Then I had to go back for therapy but they never understood anything.

In the hospital, out of 27 people there were only 7 of us who didn't smoke. We tried to stay away from the other people in a back room. To make things worse, my roommate wore perfume. The doctor finally did ask her to quit. I was really sick when I got home and I put myself back on all the stuff I was taking.

Not long after that, Dr. Penn added the Nizoral. He had treated people with AIDS so he knew that you could get candidiasis from other things besides a terminal illness. That's what the doctors first kept telling me—that I had to be terminal to have a yeast problem. I kept praying they'd find my terminal illness. I was so sick. Life wasn't any fun at all. I don't know how I dragged myself through at the time. People call me now and I can tell by their voices how tired and heavy they feel.

Then I heard about the candida conference in Memphis—I think that was the Fall of 1988—and my husband and I decided to come. I had a hard time getting there. I was very tired when we were there. I could function. In fact I never really quit functioning and go to bed or isolate myself totally. God just gave me extra strength to raise my two kids. I really lost about five years.

I have to watch what I eat. I can't eat fruit. Once in a while I'll take a section of an apple. I can't do sugar at all. I really think I was a border line diabetic years ago when they tested me. I really think I have hypoglycemia. I have to eat as soon as I get out of bed practically.

Although life is still a struggle, I don't feel tired and heavy like I used to in the 80s. I had all sorts of bladder problems when I was really sick. The doctors then gave me everything they make for vaginal yeast problems and nothing would clear it up. Then the doctor gave me nystatin for my esophagus when it was burning so bad and that medicine helped heal my vaginal problems. There were clues all along the way that what I really had was a yeast problem all over. Today my esophagus is healed and I don't have any more problems with my reflux.

I actually believe that there are a lot of older people that have reflux problems that have a severe yeast problem from all the medications they've taken and it's being totally missed. They have so many antibiotics and stuff.

I now go places but if I do some really stupid things for two or three days in a row, then I just have to stay home. The 4th of July was a really hard day for me so my husband and I stayed in. I also stay away from candles and tires in a store. A new store will undo me. It doesn't make me as sick as it used to and it doesn't take me as long to get better.

We have two children who are grown and married and two grandchildren. My husband is doing fine since he retired from the military. He's working at a factory right now doing manpower studies and stuff. He comes home in the winter time smelling so bad he really needs to find something else to do. He's probably killing himself. They paint and have a wood shop and weld and all this horrible stuff. So sometimes when he comes in he'll have to take a shower. I really have a hard time with that.

One of the doctors I've seen in the last decade is Dr. Bruce Staten of Independence, MO. He's an allergist and into environmental medicine. He told me he heard a noise in my stomach so I went and checked that out but they couldn't find anything. But he's very good in understanding environmental stuff. He's way into that.

⋘ ✉ ⋙

When Linda and her husband came to Memphis almost 13 years ago they brought me a beautiful University of Nebraska jacket. During the next year we began to correspond and I asked Linda to serve as a member of the International Health Foundation Advisory Board. Because of her experiences, kindness and compassion, she has advised and helped many people in her community and the surrounding areas with yeast problems and chemical sensitivities.

Dr. Crook

Theresa

I saw, Theresa, a woman now in her 40s, many times during her childhood and teen years. Although she experienced no serious illnesses, she was bothered by recurrent infections which at times required antibiotic drugs. During her teen years she began to be troubled by occasional vaginal yeast infections, menstrual cramps, PMS and drowsiness.

Then in her early and mid-twenties she developed additional problems, including urinary infections and more vaginal yeast infections. Theresa came in to see me in 1981. Here are excerpts from her medical records.

I fall asleep anywhere and if I don't eat at frequent intervals I become weak. I feel dizzy on getting up and at times I feel real spaced out, like I'm not on this planet. My memory's been poor and sometimes I can't even remember the names of people I know well. I feel uncoordinated, I stumble and drop things. My arms and legs ache. I'm also bothered by mood swings, frequent frontal headaches and severe menstrual cramps.

Because of the complexity of Theresa's problems, I referred her to an endocrinologist for further study and work up. And on a treatment program which included a high protein diet and supplemental vitamins, Theresa showed some improvement.

However, she continued to be bothered by recurrent vaginal yeast infections, fatigue and lethargy.

Because I'd helped a handful of my adult patients with these symptoms, I prescribed nystatin, a special diet and nutritional supplements. Although Theresa experienced a few ups and downs, she improved remarkably. When I saw her again several weeks later, she said:

I feel great. No headaches, no spaced out feelings, lots of energy, only occasional mild menstrual cramps. Life is full and exciting.

In May 2001, I called Theresa to check on how she was getting along. Here are excerpts from our conversation.

I've really done well. If I hadn't known how to treat my yeast problems, I don't know where I would be today. Except for routine check ups, I have rarely been to a doctor and I can't remember the last time I took an antibiotic. I exercise, stick to my diet and take nutritional supplements, and I keep a supply of nystatin on hand. If I start getting that yeasty feeling, I'll take nystatin for a few days and it goes away. Thank you again for the help you gave me.

SECTION THREE

Women Over 50

Alice*

Ifirst saw 42-year-old Alice† on February 19, 1977. She came in to see me because she had suffered from chronic urticaria (hives) for 3½ years. She had been studied and treated at a university medical center but found little help.

Following this hospitalization, she came to me and I worked with her for the next two years. During this time I put her in the hospital, fasted her and used various trial elimination/challenge diets and allergy tests of various sorts were carried out. Medication I gave her included prednisone, hydroxyzine hydrochloride (Atarax), hydroxyzine pamoate (Vistaril), ephedrine, terbutaline sulfate (Brethine), and cyproheptadine hydrochloride (Periactin). None of them gave her anything except temporary symptomatic help.

Alice was hospitalized again at the university medical cen-

---

*Not her real name.

†In March 1983 I published an article in the *Journal of the Tennessee Medical Association* (Vol. 76, No. 3, 1983, pp. 145–149) entitled, "The Coming Revolution in Medicine." In this article I focused on food and chemical sensitivities as a cause of chronic complaints which were affecting many patients. I also included in my Bibliography references to publications by other physicians, beginning in the 1930s.

Included in these references were three articles by C. Orian Truss, M.D., a Birmingham, Alabama, allergist and internist which were published in the *Journal of Orthomolecular Psychiatry* in 1978, 1980 and 1981. Although I learned from all of Truss' reports, I was especially impressed by his article, "The Role of *Candida albicans* in Human Illness" (J. Ortho. Psy., 10:228–238, 1981). Alice was one of the five patients I included in my 1983 article.

ter and studied further. In addition to many medications, she required twice daily injections of long-acting epinephrine to control her symptoms. The bottom line: None of Alice's studies or therapies found an answer for her recurrent hives.

In October 1979, she came back to see me. This was only a few months after I had learned about the observations of Dr. C. Orian Truss. So I prescribed nystatin (one 500,000 unit tablet four times a day), along with a yeast-free, low carbohydrate diet. **Her hives improved significantly in five days and gradually subsided over the next five months!**

Other symptoms, including rhinitis, sinusitis, fatigue and mental confusion also gradually improved, and nystatin was tapered off and then discontinued after one year. At a January 1982 follow-up visit, Alice commented, "I'm working every day. No hives. No medication. I feel great."

◄►◄► ⊠ ◄►◄►

Chronic hives is perhaps the toughest problem faced by allergists. Nystatin and antiyeast therapy do not provide a magic cure to all patients with this disorder. I saw some patients in whom it provided little help. Alice's response, plus a few reported to me by other physicians, including Dr. Robert Skinner of the University of Tennessee Department of Dermatology, make me feel that nystatin, Diflucan and a special sugar-free special diet may help some of these suffering patients.

Some years ago prominent allergists at a national convention said, "I'd rather see a tiger come into my office than a patient with chronic hives."

Dr. Crook

Ann

I was the typical poster child for candida overgrowth. I remember as a child having many colds, flus, ear infections and tubes in my ears. By the time I was nine I was immune to penicillin because I had had it so much. The antibiotics continued throughout my childhood, as well as the progression of my symptoms.

Hormonal imbalances and a weakened immune system persisted until I was 18, at which time I had my first health crisis. I was diagnosed with EBV and mononucleosis. After a couple of months of bed rest, I still wasn't any better. I began seeking out specialists and saw over eight of them, who pumped me full of more than 30 different medications, most of them antibiotics and steroids. The doctors were playing guessing games with me because everything on my tests came up negative.

As days went by I became more symptomatic and felt as though I was dying. I lost weight. I was extremely fatigued, disoriented and had intense brain fog. My chest and breathing was constriction and I was constipated. I literally was sick all over and was showing signs of leukemia. It was a year into not feeling well that I came across an alternative practitioner. She was a colon therapist. I went to see her because I had been constipated for two weeks. She was the first person that mentioned candida. I had no idea what she was talking about.

A week later, I went into a bookstore and I saw Dr. William Crook's book *The Yeast Connection*. It had just come out and it was a complete godsend. It really was. I read through it and took the questionnaire. I started to cry because I finally felt like I was validated and knew what was going on with my body.

I began a protocol of taking nystatin along with staying diligent on the candida diet. It took me a full year but then I felt healthy and whole again. What I did not understand, though, was that health entailed more than just addressing the physical body. I hadn't looked at what health meant to me on an emotional/mental level.

The other part that I did not realize was that yeast overgrowth in chronic cases can come back even more virulent if a moderate diet is not maintained. So at age 24 I was sitting in a restaurant and I had my first attack. It was like having a conscious epileptic attack. I couldn't breathe, swallow or move for about 30 seconds. My body started to spasm and tremor uncontrollably.

I went to a specialist the next day and he gave me a neurological examination and sent me off to have an EEG and evoked potential testing done. A couple of days later the doctor sat with my mother and me and said "Well the good news is you don't have cancer. The bad news is you have multiple sclerosis." I sat in shock as he suggested experimental chemotherapy drugs to try. My mother was furious at his presentation and she helped me out of his office. That was the day I walked away from Western medicine.

My case was very progressive. I had attacks daily for the

first nine months, which means immune response attacks where I was temporarily paralyzed and then my body would spasm and tremor uncontrollably. I had a near death experience three months into it. I also had 15 amalgam fillings removed without any novocaine or anesthesia because if you put anything in me, such as a needle or something invasive, I would have an attack immediately. I had two or three fillings removed at a time and became violently ill after each extraction. This process took about two to three months.

What I did to get the mercury residues out of my body was drink one to two quarts of Red Clover tea to cleanse my bloodstream, liver and kidneys. The first several months I was bedridden because of the progressive nature of my MS. I started to do some research and it took me right back to candida.

I immediately got on the candida diet and took nystatin for two years. At the end of two years I was in remission and by the next two I felt as though I'd transformed my body. In addition to taking an antifungal and cleaning up my diet, I addressed emotional and mental issues. I had suppressed anger, low self-worth and a lot of fear and realized how that played out in my illness.

I also took a little supplementation. I took Evening Primrose Oil, essential fatty acids, vitamin C, Red Clover tea and probably a couple of other things I don't remember. The supplementation was moderate but I was very diligent with my regimen. I stuck to it and by the time I was 28 I was in a new body. It has been seven years where I don't have the slightest symptom or sign of MS. It is gone.

Having a history of chronic yeast overgrowth I need to keep my yeast in check and balanced. I maintain that balance by taking an herbal antifungal in a low dose each day. I'm also moderate with my diet. I eat as I would on a candida diet Monday through Friday and on the weekends I eat what I want. I also take vitamins/minerals, essential fatty acids and amino acids to keep my immune system functioning optimally. On those occasions of vacations and holidays I will drink one quart of Red Clover tea and increase my antifungal when I return home for about a week to clean myself out.

A couple of years after my illness it became obvious that I wanted to help others get healthy. Today I am a Naturopathic Doctor and Clinical Hypnotherapist. I have a private practice in West Hollywood, California and specialize in candida, allergies, gastrointestinal disorders, hormonal imbalances and autoimmune diseases. I am also an inspirational speaker and educator and have written a book, *How To Cure Multiple Sclerosis*. This book is available on my website, www.annboroch.com.

I have had many successes from mild conditions to so-called incurable diseases. My first patient was cured of fibromyalgia which had yeast overgrowth as the primary cause. I look at a person's body/mind/spirit, which allows me to get to the core of their imbalances. From there I use many natural integrative techniques, such as nutritional therapy, herbs, vitamins, detoxification methods and work with the subconscious mind. I feel my success comes from how I examine the body as a whole and how I empower my patients by educating them.

⋙ ⊠ ⋘

Ann and I began to correspond about a year ago. In February 2001 she came from Los Angeles over to Anaheim to visit me. I was impressed and am still impressed by what she has been doing, and continues to do.

Dr. Crook

Buddy and Carol Young

Between February 1, 2000, and June 8, 2001, I received four beautifully written letters from W. R. "Buddy" Young of Waco, Texas. There were 31 pages in all and the story Buddy tells is clearly expressed, interesting, convincing, heartbreaking, yet encouraging. Reading his letters also shows his wonderful love for his wife, his courage and his persistence in spite of seeming overwhelming odds. Here now are excerpts from Buddy's letters.

February 1, 2000:

To the Administrator, International Health Foundation.
PLEASE SEND INFO A.S.A.P.

Please send me the list of physicians and the package of information on yeast and fungus-related disorders. I suspect my wife, Carol, may have a very serious yeast-related illness.

In Feb. of 1999 Carol had some small pimple-like eruptions appear on her head. She asked the doctor to give her something to heal it.

The doctor wrote a prescription for topical Clindamycin. The eruptions began to spread to her arm. The doctor prescribed a broad spectrum antibiotic CEPHALEXIN orally to take in conjunction while continuing to use the topical

CLINDAMYCIN. The infection continued to worsen and spread to other parts of her body.

Over a period of nine months she was on daily doses of Cephalexin, Clindamycin, Cefadroxil and tetracycline. During this time the eruptions spread over her entire body except for the soles of her feet and the genital area. She had break outs on her scalp which I can only describe as boggy, oozing sores. The hair follicle seems to have died and the hair does not grow back.

The eruptions on her body are about the same size diameter of a small pencil eraser. They start with a small blister which bursts within a few hours of appearing and they begin to swell and ooze a white cheesy substance, then they begin to bleed. After 8 or 9 months of this condition worsening her doctor said she should see a dermatologist but did not refer us to one. We called around and was told by most they were not taking any new patients. We finally found one to look at my wife at the family practice clinic. He looked at my wife, shrugged his shoulders and said, "I don't have any idea what it is." Then he charged us $120.

My wife's symptoms worsened. The sites of the eruptions are painful. Her joints have began to swell. She has developed edema in her legs and arms. It is now painful for her to walk or get in or out of bed. Carol had worsened to a point that I took her back to our family clinic late one evening in October 1999. I told the doctor my pharmacist had said the problem may be caused by the antibiotics over a 9 month period. I had also mentioned this to my wife's regular doctor. The reply was, "No WAY."

I'd read several books which I found in the medical

section of the public library on the subject of systemic infections caused by antibiotics. I begged the doctor to write a prescription for nystatin, which she reluctantly did. After taking nystatin for a few days the sores began to heal. The scalp also began to heal. When the nystatin was gone I called for a refill. The doctor did not respond.

After five days without the medicine my wife had a full relapse of all symptoms. I again called the doctor's office and talked with the nurse and related to her what had happened. She said she would have the doctor call in the refill. It was not refilled. By this time the office was closed.

I called the emergency number and told the doctor on call what was going on. He said he saw no reason not to refill the Rx and called it in again. After a few days my wife's condition began to improve. She was feeling much better and healing. I again asked for a refill and it was refused. After several days again my wife had a full relapse. I again begged for a refill and it was finally filled. This time the condition did not respond as well as before.

My wife is very ill! From what I've been able to gather by reading medical books and the information given to me by the pharmacist, she has all the symptoms of a systemic yeast infection and the suppressed immune system symptoms: Fatigue, Lethargy, Depression, Inability to concentrate, Feeling spacey or disconnected, Headaches, Skin problems, Joint pain/swelling, Vaginal discharge, Poor coordination, cramps, abdominal pain, Diarrhea, Bloating, Edema, Muscle cramps, weakness, Lowered (NO) Sex drive and a general feeling of serious illness.

From what I've read this condition can become life threatening and I am very concerned. Last Feb. my wife went to the doctor for treatment of a minor skin problem and ended up with a serious illness. What is amazing to me is the uncaring attitude of the doctors we've seen, and the seeming unwillingness to look at the documented material that I've gathered from the medical literature written by the A.M.A., Columbia Medical School, University of Texas Health Science Center, etc. I have also read books by William G. Crook, M.D., Orian Truss, M.D., and John Parks Trowbridge, M.D.

The sad thing to me is we've received virtually no help from doctors we've seen. Been given no referrals. Have encountered the attitude of "don't bother me with this problem, I don't know anything about this illness and don't have time to learn about it." The only person who has helped us is a pharmacist who gave us material from pharmaceutical companies and encouraged me to search the medical literature for help.

The International Health Foundation was recommended in a book by William G. Crook, M.D., in his 1986 book on yeast connected illnesses, and I'm enclosing a check for $25 as recommended in the book. Please send me the information packet and list as soon as possible.

Walker R. Young
Waco, Texas

In another long letter received by the International Health Foundation, Mr. Young summarizes his wife's history. Here are excerpts.

June 15, 2000:

I thank God for doctors like Dr. William G. Crook and Dr. Orian Truss. Doctors who, regardless of criticism, are willing to stand on the cutting edge; doctors who don't get bogged down on the popular medical establishment blindly following the old ways while ignoring the new; doctors who are willing to read a letter pleading for help because the person writing has a loved one who is slowly dying from a doctor-caused illness and can find no one to listen to them. Dr. Crook, you and others like you have earned a place in medical history. A place of greatness because you care! You took your valuable time to read my letter, call my home, speak to me about my wife's illness, then send me the names of caring doctors. Because of you my wife is on the road to recovery.

Dr. Ted Edwards said Carol had the worst systemic candida infection he'd ever seen. Dr. Crook, again, let me thank you for saving my wife's life. I'm also thankful to live in a country where information is available to the general public. Unless I was able to obtain this information from my public library, my wife might not be alive today. It took an uncaring and ignorant doctor nine months, 253–500 mg tablets and 240 ml of topical broad spectrum antibiotics to make my wife seriously ill. It will take 1–2 years to get her well.

After several months of treatment with Diflucan, olive leaf extract, flaxseed oil, Lactobacillus and plenty of rest, she's shown great improvement. Her skin eruptions, edema and swollen lymph nodes are gone and her interest in everyday life is returning. She'll be scarred from the lesions for the rest of her life, but at least she will have her health. She's still having problems with swollen joints which are very painful. She must rest much more than before this illness, but the bottom line is she is recovering.

I could write 100 pages and still not tell you the whole story. I'll close by telling you that you may use any information I send you if you feel it will help educate other physicians or help others. Thank you again.

Walker R. "Buddy" Young, Jr.
Waco, TX

PS—This is not much, but I'm enclosing a $10 donation to IHF and will keep sending more donations in the future. Keep up the good work.

March 20, 2001:

Dr. Crook,

I hope things are well with you. You asked me to keep you updated on my wife's condition. It has been some time since I've written. My wife, Carol, and myself (Walker R. Young), most folks call me "Buddy," are so grateful to you for letting the world know about the problems *Candida albicans* can cause. If you can't remember who we are, I'm the person in Waco, Texas who wrote you a letter and asked for help for my wife, who had been given large doses of broad spectrum antibiotics for nine months by a physician. This doctor has a problem of not wanting to listen to her patients.

We started seeing a doctor who was on the list sent to us by the International Health Foundation. At the time I contacted you my wife was almost totally bedfast she was so ill. She was given Diflucan, as you recommended, she took it for three months after being diagnosed with "the worst case of systemic candidiasis" this doctor had ever seen. All of her sores, ulcers and lesions were completely healed within a month and a half, with the exception of the large oozing places on her scalp. They did get better.

She was taken off Diflucan after three months and put on nystatin. The majority of her symptoms were much better. Then two months ago she started having edema in her legs and ankles again and some of her former symptoms returned. I took her back to see the P.A.C. in Austin last week because her lower legs had swollen to about twice the normal size and she was so tired all the time. She has a hard time doing anything.

Four days ago I convinced the P.A.C. to put her back on Diflucan. Since starting this medication, as of this writing, her legs and ankles have started to go down, although the lack of energy and depression are still present. We've been told it may take three to five years for a complete recovery. She's taking 100 mg of Diflucan daily and I can see improvement in this short time.

The doctor seems very hesitant about using Diflucan longer than a couple of months, but it seems to work miracles when she's taking it. She's also taking olive leaf extract along with antifungals and I'm doing the cooking and trying to follow the recommended diet. If you have any suggestions other than what we're doing for her illness we would appreciate your advice. Again let me thank you for your kindness and help. I will tell anyone who will listen about the International Health Foundation. I'm enclosing a check for $30 to help with your work.

Thanks again

Walker "Buddy" R. Young

PS—Keep telling doctors to listen to their patients. My wife would never have become so ill had her doctor just taken time to listen!!!

June 8, 2001:

In this letter Buddy Young, a retired sprinkler/pipe fitter, said that he has concern for his hard-working associates who, by their labor have "made this world a healthier, safer place to live." He also reviewed the 13 different prescriptions for broad-spectrum antibiotics given to Carol between February 1, 1999 and October 4, 1999.

He also described efforts he went through for over a year to find another doctor. He said, "I just wanted my wife to get well." The doctor told me, "Your wife has a nervous rash."

Then he said,

As I told you in my last letter, Carol's symptoms were slowly returning after the Diflucan was discontinued. On Carol's next visit I took your letter concerning the long term use of Diflucan, and after a blood profile was done, Carol was put back on Diflucan. She's again improving . . . The remaining problems she has are 1. On her scalp in the area where she lost her hair due to the infection . . . 2. She still has problems with low energy. She seems to need much more sleep than normal . . . 3. At times the depression returns but it then goes away.

Her memory has greatly improved and she even has begun to read at times. It's been a slow process but she's very much improved over a year ago. At that time she was so ill she never got out of the house . . . Believe me she's improved so much it seems like a miracle to me . . . Thank you Billy for your continued interest. I feel as if I've known you for all of my life. You remind me of the doctor I had as a child who thought nothing of coming to our house to take care of my big toe when I almost cut it off. I will close now because I could ramble on about the medical experiences of the past 20 years. I have your new book, *Tired—So Tired!*, although I've only glanced through it so far. Thanks again for your help. I'm enclosing a small donation for the International Health Foundation."

Buddy Young

＊＊＊ ✉ ＊＊＊

Re-reading all of Buddy Young's 31-page story made me feel it should be included in this book. What he had to say made me more determined to bring the yeast connection story into the medical mainstream. I can understand the desire of my fellow physicians to look for more "scientific proof" of the yeast connection. Yet, if they will take time from their busy, busy schedules and listen to people like Buddy Young, they'll be able to help many more of their patients.

Dr. Crook

Dorothy

In the late 1960s—I'm not sure of the exact date—I began to be troubled with urinary infections. Although my urinary symptoms would usually go away when my doctor gave me antibiotics or sulfa drugs, my symptoms kept coming back. They did some x-rays and other tests which showed that kidney stones were the reason I kept having problems. My doctor put me on a sulfa drug, which I took every day for seven years.

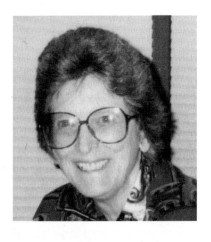

If I didn't take it I got a kidney or bladder infection. I got to where my skin just smelled like sulfur. Then I passed those two stones and I quit taking the sulfa.

In the mid-1970s I noticed that I was losing strength. My head hurt most of the time and I had problems with my vision that would come and go. I was also bothered by joint pains. These symptoms, too, would come and go. I was able to keep on working, but I seemed to get weaker each year. In 1980 an eye doctor said I had scars in both eyes and in 1981 my left eye went out. The doctor said it was optic neuritis. He also told me that I probably had MS.

They did all sorts of tests on me, but they didn't show anything. Although my eye symptoms got better, I got to where I was falling and I had what I call "electricity" running around in my legs. I felt they had something clamped on them and I couldn't get it off. It hurt so bad at times I felt like I'd scream if I couldn't get out of my legs. I felt like a person with boots on who needed to take them off. I also felt drugged and weak.

Then when I brought my daughter, Ann, to see you, you asked me how I was and I told you some of my symptoms. You said you thought you might be able to help me. You started me on the yeast-free, sugar-free diet, nystatin, vitamins and minerals. But when I started taking the nystatin powder it made everything worse. I stuck with it and experimented with the dose and gradually my symptoms got better. After a while I shifted over to tablets and took them every day. I stayed on my diet strictly for four and a half years. I didn't even have anything in my house I shouldn't eat.

Then the last year of staying on the diet that strict, I was also off anything gluten. At that point, both big toes were numb and I had some numb places on the side of my leg by my knee. I stayed on that gluten-free diet for six months and the numbness went away—and is still gone. That was in 1989.

Now I eat pretty much what I want. I do watch anything with yeast in it. If I eat bread with yeast I can tell. It does something to me. It makes my insides not feel right and I get tingling in my legs. So I just don't eat it. I still take the vitamins and nystatin, but I don't take it all the time. I just take it morning and night, two tablets. Then if I eat something during the day I shouldn't I'll take it at night too. When I'm off it for a while I can tell I need to take it back. My insides feel bloated and I just don't feel good. And when I start taking it I feel better. My body adjusts.

I know that prayer helped me too. I've always been a person who turns to the Lord and prays because I have a brother with cerebral palsy and my mother read the Bible to him and we prayed. It was just part of my life. And I asked the Lord for help. I'd read in the scripture how he heals folks. I really believe that the way he answered was in the coming to the place of understanding of what was going on in my body. And then getting to you and you telling me what to do.

I kept on working and I was going to retire when I was 62, but when I got to that age I decided to go ahead and work. That went on for about three more years and I got to be 65 and I thought, well I'll retire. Then they signed the bill about drawing SS and work as much as I wanted to so I thought I would do that. And I'm continuing to work.

I go to all the health departments in West Tennessee (20 counties) every other month to each one. I have ten health departments a month that I go to. What I do is I carry my equipment (which weighs 15 lbs each), a portable audiometer and a tympanometer, and check hearing. If their hearing is okay I tell them that it is. If it's not okay then I refer them to a medical doctor, an ENT or an audiologist to get what they need. This is what I do. Then I have office duties also. I work for the State Health Department and I work out of the regional office here in Jackson. My title is speech and hearing assistant. We do speech screening, but not much since the educational department has taken that over from age 3.

I rarely have that concrete feeling in my legs anymore. Not more than once a year. It seems to me it happens when I haven't taken my medicine like I should or I've been eating something I shouldn't. I'll correct it and it goes away. I take Basic Preventive #5, vitamin C, calcium, magnesium, B12, garlic, Co-Q$_{10}$, grapeseed extract, niacin amide, lecithin granules, acidophilus and flax seed oil. I haven't been back to the neurologist in a long time. Last time I went was when I had that last spell with the optic neuritis. Dr James Spruill did an MRI and found no plaque. That was 5 years ago.

Then my Jackson eye doctor sent me to Memphis to Dr. Richard Drewery. He did all kinds of tests and he told me that people who have optic neuritis either have MS or will have it. And he told me at that point my eye was beginning to come back. This is when my right eye went completely out. Since then I've gotten it back, not completely, but it's okay for reading and driving. The sun hurts my eyes. I don't read as much as I used to because the blind spots interfere. I can read and I can do my job and drive.

I am thankful for the answer to my prayers, which led me to you and the diet, and nystatin, vitamins, minerals and other supplements. I feel like if I hadn't gotten on the yeast-free, sugar-free diet and on the nystatin and vitamins and minerals that I would be in a wheelchair now. And when I think back to where I was headed I couldn't function today because it was moving fast. But it stopped. It took a while and I had to be really rigid about the diet and the medicine. I used to think I could never stay on a diet but I did and it helped me and I'm so thankful.

✳✳✳ ✉ ✳✳✳

I included part of Dorothy's story in the first edition of **The Yeast Connection** *which was published in 1983, in the 1986 paperback edition of that book and in* **The Yeast Connection and the Woman** *published in 1995 and 1998.*

Because I learned from friends that Dorothy was doing well and still working, I called her in May 2001 and recorded our conversation. Her story is an important one for several reasons.

- ◇ *It documents the importance of multiple therapies, including antifungal medication, dietary changes, avoidance of foods that cause sensitivity reactions, the use of nutritional supplements and prayer.*
- ◇ *It shows that the person with a yeast-related problem often experiences ups and downs.*
- ◇ *It shows courage.*
- ◇ *It also shows clearly that persistence and staying the course can help a person overcome a serious and often devastating health problem.*

Dr. Crook

Ebony*

first saw 33-year-old Ebony† on July 10, 1982. She came in with a whole "laundry list" of complaints including dizziness, nausea, nasal congestion, night cough, chest pain, bladder symptoms and premenstrual tension. Here are excerpts from her history, written in her own words:

I'm ready to find out if it's all in my head or whether it's something really making me sick. All my childhood I suffered with stomach problems which were usually blamed on nerves. Several years ago, I developed a strange swelling in my ankles and feet which kept me from walking for several weeks. About the same time . . . in the fall of 1980 . . . I began having headaches, dizziness, nausea, sore throat and earaches. Antihistamines and antibiotics helped a little.

---

*Not her real name.

†In March 1983 I published an article in the *Journal of the Tennessee Medical Association* (Vol. 76, No. 3, 1983, pp. 145–149) entitled, "The Coming Revolution in Medicine." In this article I focused on food and chemical sensitivities as a cause of chronic complaints which were affecting many patients. I also included in my Bibliography references to publications by other physicians, beginning in the 1930s.

Included in these references were three articles by C. Orian Truss, M.D., a Birmingham, Alabama allergist and internist which were published in the *Journal of Orthomolecular Psychiatry* in 1978, 1980 and 1981. Although I learned from all of Truss' reports, I was especially impressed by his article, "The Role of *Candida albicans* in Human Illness." (J. Ortho. Psy., 10:228–238, 1981.) Ebony was one of the five patients I included in my 1983 article.

Food elimination helped to some degree but I continued to be troubled by persistent night cough.

Then, after a short exposure to paint, I felt sick with generalized aching. Also, I developed peculiar symptoms following injections of Novocain by the dentist, including confusion, fatigue, and light-headedness. In the spring of 1982, 1 developed bladder problems, including infections, frequent urination, and incomplete evacuation of my bladder.

Ebony's general physical examination was non-revealing except for dark infraorbital circles and an overall appearance of fatigue. Allergy testing to common inhalants showed no reactions. I started her on 1 million units of nystatin four times a day and a yeast-free diet. Ebony began improving within ten days after being started on the treatment program.

In a November 1982 follow-up visit, Ebony said,

Dr. Crook, thank you for your help. The treatment program you designed for me has really made a difference. But if I cheat on my diet or leave off my nystatin, many of my symptoms begin coming back. So I'm more careful about my diet and I continue the nystatin. If I'm not improving as fast as I would like I'll up my doses of nystatin to 2,000,000 units four times a day.

•• •• •• ✉ •• •• ••

Ebony moved away in 1983 and although I've tried to track her down to get an updated report, I have been unsuccessful.

Dr. Crook

Judith

I first became ill in 1970 following a bad case of flu. Instead of all recovering normally I continued to deteriorate and the unexplained illness kept me in bed for six months. A string of doctors insisted that since my tests were all normal, I was not physically ill, and suggested psychiatric care. Eventually I returned, rather shakily, to work.

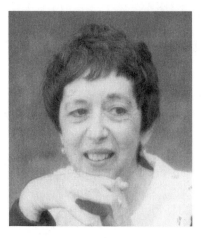

I assumed that this strange episode was just a fluke, a one-time event that I could put behind me.

It was not to be. The illness that had no name returned again and again, throwing my life into utter disarray. Eighteen years passed as I became sick and then well, and then sick again. I spent a lot of time trapped in bed, wondering how such a devastating disease could be totally dismissed by the medical profession. Even during "well"periods I didn't feel normal; I experienced distortions in my senses of sight, hearing and taste. I also noticed strange reactions to all sorts of chemicals, which grew steadily worse.

In 1988, as you know, the CDC was forced to recognize

this condition due to the increasing number of patients. The official name they chose, Chronic Fatigue Syndrome, was a wastebasket term with little meaning, but I was grateful for the validation and hopeful that research would produce a cure.

However, I was dismayed by the fact that researchers were concentrating on finding a viral cause for the disease. It seemed that "new" viruses were all the rage, new diseases were appearing, and virologists were eagerly trying to match them all up. But in my experience, this illness didn't behave like a viral infection at all. For one thing, it usually affected random individuals rather than groups. For another, it had a preference for females. Viruses, as far as I knew, couldn't tell the difference between girls and boys. And it tended to strike at young adults, normally the healthiest and most disease-resistant segment of the population. How then could it be caused by a contagious bug?

I let myself be treated for viruses such as EBV, but with no results; my health continued to decline. Finally, in 1989, I collapsed at work. Somehow I made my way home to bed, where I remained for the next five years. I could barely crawl from the bedroom to the bathroom, and only survived because my husband took care of me—his life, I feared, had become even more difficult than mine.

At one point, to minimize my exposure to allergens (our old Victorian house was full of them), I moved to a small room in Berkeley. I couldn't bear the chemical smells that visitors brought with them, so with the exception of visits from my husband and very occasional others, I lived for a year in solitary confinement.

Even that didn't stop my inexorable downward slide. I weighed about 80 pounds. My digestive process—not to mention my mental faculties—seemed to have shut down for good. I was in severe pain, and my allergies exploded to include almost every chemical imaginable. Exposure to ordinary things like books, newspapers, TV, or plastic bags set my brain reeling. A constant "brain fog" dogged me.

And then, unexpectedly, I was diagnosed at last—not by seeing a doctor, but by talking on the phone to a nutritionist. I learned that I probably had severe systemic candidiasis. Not long after, the diagnosis was confirmed when I looked into my mouth. To my horror, I saw a veritable rain forest of white gummy growth hanging in strings off the edges of my tongue. The mystery malady was solved at last. I should mention at this point that there were multiple factors involved in causing me to become so severely fungus-ridden, beyond the usual culprits of birth control pills, antibiotics and moldy environment. I worked for years as an artist/printmaker, practically bathing in dangerous printing chemicals. There's no doubt in my mind that these toxic substances, and not any virus, were the root of my illness.

With the problem identified, I was able to assemble and (allergies permitting) read some important books on the subject. A friend brought me "The Yeast Connection" to begin. What a relief to see it all spelled out for me! I had a real illness, it wasn't psychological, and it could be treated.

But in my case, I wondered if it might be too late. I was by this time more dead than alive—a skeleton with a heartbeat. When I became allergic even to my little Berkeley room, I was brought home, presumably to die.

Fate intervened, and almost by accident I was put in contact with a doctor who understood this condition and how to treat it, Dr. Vincent Marinkovich. Under his care I began a program of diet and antifungal drugs—which for long periods of time caused me severe and constant die-off reactions. I didn't care—those reactions meant that I was on the right track at last.

One day, more than a year after I began treatment, I embarked on a great adventure. I left the house under my own power and went for a walk. A very slow walk to be sure, but most exciting. I was out in the world again!

My struggle, now three decades long, has been painful but has taught me some wonderful lessons. It tried my will to survive and showed that will to be more resilient than I expected. It tested my husband's love and caring for me, and that, too, proved to be stronger and deeper than I knew. It taught me the absolute necessity of thinking for myself, for I had to defy the doctors and search elsewhere for the real cause of my illness—the cause that has such profound implications not only for me, but for the lives of others as well.

••••• ✉ •••••

Judith Lopez and I began to correspond in the spring of 1999. She sent me the manuscript of her book. I read it, I liked what she said and encouraged her to publish it. I was pleased when she followed through and she sent me an autographed copy. The book is entitled **IMMUNE DYSFUNCTION—Winning**

My Battle Against Toxins, Illness & the Medical Establishment.*

I love the book and I sent her these comments: As riveting as a novel that you can't put down. This provocative memoir will provide help and hope to countless people—especially those who experience devastating fatigue, unexplained aches and pains, chemical sensitivities, memory problems, accompanying depression and a feeling of being sick all over . . . Comprehensive and authoritative . . . I give it my highest recommendation.

Dr. Crook

---

*This book is available from Millpond Press, P.O. Box 2524, Mill Valley, CA 94942; www.bookzone.com; www.amazon.com and at 800-852-4890.

Karen

T his 31-year-old registered nurse and mother first came to see me in 1981. Because her history illustrates so many important issues, I'm including most of a letter she sent me a year later.

As a child, I took many unneeded antibiotics for colds and well-meaning neighbors provided me with too much candy. Knowing what I know now, I feel both of these factors set the stage for my long battle with vaginal problems.

Trouble with menstrual cramps began when I started my period at age 12. But after my first yeast infection at age 17, my cramps became severe enough to spend a day in bed every month. And during the week before each period, I was irritable, bloated and generally miserable.

I began on birth control pills a month before my marriage at age 19. I took them for three months, but felt so bad I had to discontinue them. I promptly became pregnant and was bothered by cystitis and vaginal yeast infections throughout my pregnancy.

The next 2½ years brought two more pregnancies, one of which was spontaneously aborted. During this time I was treated with antibiotics for 10 episodes of "cystitis." Recently, my doctor commented, *"Many of your symptoms were probably caused by candida irritation of your bladder outlet . . . the urethra."*

I also experienced joint pains and swelling, involving especially my knees. And I was given cortisone and other steroids on several occasions. I began to notice, for the first time, that getting around odorous cleaning materials made me sick.

Then early in my third pregnancy, I had my first migraine headache and I had no idea that it could be related to diet and my other problems.

After the birth of my second child, I took birth control pills for seven months, but once again I had to stop them because I felt worse than I'd ever felt in my life. My vaginitis continued and my cystitis was so severe my gynecologist sent me to a urologist.

I was put on a broad-spectrum antibiotic for six weeks and told to take them anytime I had urgency and frequency for several days.

At the age of 25, my migraine headaches became so severe that I consulted a neurosurgeon. Various drugs were prescribed to control the migraines. Yet these drugs caused so many side effects and so much emotional upset that I soon stopped them. About that time, because of my persistent vaginal problems, I went to a gynecologist. Although he was kind during my first visit, he finally lost his patience and told me not to "bother" him with something as unimportant as vaginal infections! He told me I'd have to learn to live with them.

My fourth pregnancy at age 26 put more pressure on what I now realize was my weakened immune system. I was given progesterone for an irritable uterus and while I was taking it my vaginal problems were aggravated. And as I've since learned, pregnancy also worsens vaginal yeast problems.

I went into labor at around 32 weeks and was given intravenous alcohol and steroids. Soon afterward, I experienced severe burning in my throat, esophagus and stomach which lasted for 5 months and kept me depressed and very uncomfortable. I also experienced visual disturbances, along with abdominal bloating and constipation. My fatigue was full-blown by now, but I attributed it to having a new baby. I also noticed that turning on the gas heat that winter triggered my migraine headaches.

Although during my fifth pregnancy, at age 27, I ate plenty of good foods, I craved sweets and junk foods. My visual disturbances, fatigue and vaginal problems were all prominent during this pregnancy. However, after the baby was born, I began eating a high protein, low carbohydrate diet which temporarily relieved some of my symptoms.

Then at the age of 28, all of my previous symptoms either returned or became more prominent and I experienced many new ones, including headache and severe abdominal pain. This pain was so bad that my husband took me to the doctor on two occasions because he thought I had appendicitis.

In the meantime, my ability to concentrate decreased, my memory became worse and I got up every morning tired. My vaginal symptoms of pain, burning, itching and heavy discharge were full-blown. I was taking antibiotics all the time as well as using different vaginal creams and suppositories. Nothing helped me and I became increasingly miserable.

My depression became a real problem and I cried so easily for seemingly no reason, and my premenstrual tension became worse. My husband was very supportive and that helped. He would assure me that I wasn't "crazy." (Now that I'm better, he commented recently, "I really thought I was going to lose you.")

My gynecologist was kind and tried everything he knew to do. I hate to admit it now, but some days the thought of death was pleasant. The only thing that helped me get through many days was memorizing the Psalms of the Bible. As I cried, I'd quote the scriptures and I'd get hope to go on.

At the age of 29, 1 had a hysterectomy. Some of my backache and abdominal pain improved for a while, and the premenstrual symptoms were gone. However, other symptoms developed, including numbness and tingling of my extremities, daily visual problems, excessive intestinal gas and throat mucus, joint pain and heart palpitations.

I kept a headache that never left. Sometimes it was mild, at other times it was severe. I felt so horrible I would pray, "Lord, Jesus, how can I keep living this way?" My gynecologist continued to be supportive, but I never told him of my many symptoms for fear he'd send me to a psychiatrist.

Then in October, 1981, through a sort of unique coincidence (it was definitely an answer to my prayers), I first learned about yeast-related illness. Soon afterward, I was put on a comprehensive treatment program to help me get rid of candida, improve my immune system and regain my health. Many different things have helped me, including nystatin, Nizoral and the yeast-free, low carbohydrate diet. Allergy vaccines for inhalants, foods and candida have also been essential parts of my treatment program. I've also been helped by nutritional supplements, including essential fatty acids, minerals and vitamins.

Today, November 19, 1982, my vaginal symptoms are better but they are still present and bothersome. However, all the other problems are gone all or most of the time. I feel better than I have in many years and I'm grateful for the answer to my prayers.

Karen came in for a review visit on December 21. 1982. She commented,

I'm slowly getting better, but I still have my "ups and downs." Nystatin douches help my vaginitis, but the symptoms never go away and I must take tremendous doses of nystatin to control them . . . the equivalent of 48 to 50 tablets a day. I wish I could take Nizoral again, it really helped last year. My candida shots in the weak dilutions help most of the time and I take them two or three times a week.

I continued Karen on the same basic program with a few modifications and changes. Because her liver enzymes had returned to normal, I added a small dose of Nizoral to her treatment program . . . ¼ tablet twice a week. Mold cultures of her home showed that the mold, hormodendrum, was the principle offender. Appropriate changes were then made in Karen's extracts.

During our office visit in February 1983 Karen commented,

I was involved in an automobile accident in January. I received many bruises and had to have a lot of x-rays. Although I experienced no serious injuries, I've been worse since the accident. I've had more vaginal burning and my fatigue level is high again. I was also troubled by a rash on two different days last week.

After reviewing Karen's treatment program, I made several changes. Karen returned for a follow-up visit with me in March. Here are a few of her comments.

That automobile accident really set me back. My vaginitis continues to bother me and my fatigue level remains high. My prescription for amphotericin B was filled by a French pharmacy and sent to me a couple of weeks ago.

Then in a follow-up phone report two weeks later, Karen reported,

I'm improving and I've finally gotten back to where I was before my accident in January. My fatigue and joint pains are better although on damp days when the mold count is high, I don't feel as good. I'm continuing the oral and vaginal amphotericin B. I dump the contents of 1 capsule in my mouth four times daily and insert the powder from 1 capsule into my vagina twice daily. This seems to work better than nystatin in doses of over a teaspoon of powder four times daily.

I'm also following all of the other parts of the comprehensive program of management you prescribed, including inhalant and food vaccines, flaxseed oil, primrose oil and other nutritional supplements. I also have restricted my diet to meats, eggs and vegetables for the past 10 days.

So to repeat, I'm really doing well with all symptoms except the vulvovaginitis which continues to cause varying degrees of discomfort and frustration.

In January 1984, Karen reported that she was free of vaginal pain and discomfort most of the time and that she felt great, had lots of energy and none of the other symptoms she used to have unless she cheated on her diet. She also said she couldn't tolerate perfumes, chemicals or mold exposure.

During the 1980s and early 1990s, I saw Karen many times. She also appeared with me on WHBQ-TV in Memphis and a staff member of the Canadian Broadcasting System accompanied me to Karen's home about 50 miles south of Memphis.

In June 1993 Karen told me that the severe vaginal problems which tormented her for so many years had gone away—almost as though the problem never existed. She also said,

I haven't had to take nystatin, amphotericin B, Nizoral or other oral antifungal therapy for over four years. Yet, I do notice some itching and burning during the spring and fall pollen seasons. I believe you told me it was a form of "vaginal hay fever."

Several years ago I was tormented by urinary frequency and I had to urinate up to 60 times a day. Comprehensive examinations by a urologist, plus my home diet detective work, showed that the cause was an allergic cystitis. And the medication I was taking had a corn base and I am clearly sensitive to corn in any form.

I was also sensitive to ordinary wheat bread. Through networking I found that I can tolerate whole living wheat, which is organically grown, and this enables me to have bread which I normally could not tolerate. I also take big doses of vitamin C and calcium and magnesium and take supplemental vitamins at times when I can afford them.

But compared to my health fifteen years ago, my problems are literally nonexistent. I do have a sensitive bladder and have to urinate frequently, but I drink lots of fluid.

Karen and I continued to correspond and talk on the phone, and in a conversation with me in January 1998, she said in effect,

My health is superb. And except for mild seasonal hay fever, I have no complaints. I'm delighted to know that you've included my story in *The Yeast Connection and the Woman*. It should give other women hope.

In 1999 and 2000, like many people with yeast-related problems, Karen told me of her ups and downs. She told me that she was experiencing severe chronic fatigue and other problems. In late December 2000, I prescribed thyroid medication and other measures to help her cope.

In March 2001 I recommended East Park olive leaf extract. In her April 2001 letter Karen gave me an update. Here are excerpts.

I am better and do attribute at least 95% of it to the Olive Leaf tablets, or d-Lenolate as the East Park folks refer to it. I definitely had "kill off" for 10–12 days but even in some of those times had some energy increases at times. Since then I've had a new sense of well-being as well as increased energy and much less muscle burning.

I'm by no means symptom-free, but things are definitely on the upswing. Thank you for your love, support, help and for contacting East Park on my behalf. What a blessing you are to me!!!

Although Karen improved, she continued to be troubled by persistent fatigue and I prescribed tiny doses of cortisol. In June 2001, Karen wrote and said,

I am THRILLED to report that I have seen remarkable results with just 6 weeks of cortisol!! My muscles and joints feel good, I have a new sense of well-being that has been absent for over 2½ years, my energy level is consistently higher and I'm sleeping much better.

People are telling me that they see a new spring in my step and that I look younger. THANK YOU for your encouragement to give the cortisol a trial.

Here are excerpts from my July 2001 phone visit with Karen.

I started the cortisol about six weeks ago and I feel better now than I've felt in about three years. People I talk to infrequently tell me now when I leave messages or they hear my voice in person they can tell that I'm stronger. I have a greater sense of well-being. I'm sleeping better . . . I'm walking 4 miles a day, even in this heat.

I don't have muscle aches or burning any more . . . My skin is healthier . . . My fingernails are even stronger and look different. Apparently I just had some adrenal insufficiency and cortisol seems to be the answer.

I'm also taking many supplements, including a B complex, magnesium, calcium, grapeseed extract, vitamin C, acidophilus and many others.

◆◆◆ ⊠ ◆◆◆

Because Karen was one of my first patients with yeast-related problems, her story is exciting, gratifying and much, much more.

Dr. Crook

Margaret

My complaints included extreme fatigue, drowsiness, heart palpitations, numbness in my lower legs and a feeling of tension on the sides of my neck. After my doctor made several tests, he said, "Margaret, I feel the Epstein-Barr Virus may be making you sick— or a form of mononucleosis."

My headaches were so severe I used an ice bag to try to get relief. Also I would sleep straight through the night for ten hours and then I could not stay awake the next day no matter how hard I tried. My muscles were so tender I could not stand to be touched.

Life was miserable and I started to search for answers and for help. Many different diagnoses were considered, including MS, Lupus, and even TB. All of the tests were negative. He finally diagnosed me with Chronic Fatigue Syndrome (CFS), which was just getting its name at that time. He also said I had fibromyalgia.

My condition continued to worsen until I could not talk on the phone for more than five minutes. To just walk outside took major effort. When I went to the store I had to go in a wheelchair. I could not do my housework or even cook, much less grocery shop. I had severe spells of being unable to breathe, feeling as each breath would be my last. My eyes would run, and other times I would develop an instant head cold, accompanied by hoarseness. The fatigue was sometimes so severe that I could not get out of bed no matter how bad I wanted to.

Before this came on me I was a very happy woman who loved taking care of my home, babysitting my granddaughter and being involved in my church. I love life and love people and I had always tried to make the best of any situation.

My personal physician is kind and caring and knew of my positive attitude. In an effort to help me he gave me a prescription for Prozac because he felt I was getting depressed from the months of being so sick and not finding help. I chose not to have it filled. I have a strong faith in God and had many people praying for me. I never lost faith that the answers were out there.

I started an all-out search by getting family and friends to purchase books for me on CFS. I lay in bed and read, trusting God to lead me to the right information.

Many, many months later I read a newspaper article which talked about food allergies and how they could affect a person's body. Then I came across a 1990 book about chronic fatigue which included the observations of Dr. Carol Jessop, then a professor at the University of California in San Francisco, who said that chronic fatigue was often yeast-connected.

Soon after reading this book my husband drove me to Norfolk, Virginia, for a routine visit with my physician. After this I asked him to go to a bookstore and see if there were any new books on CFS and I know this was an answer to a prayer.

In the store (which I was too sick to enter), my husband ran into a woman from our own community. He began telling her my story and she suggested the book that had really helped her. Its title, *The Yeast Connection* by Dr. William Crook. The Tidewater area is huge and for her to be in this particular store at that particular time was a small miracle.

And after reading this book, I felt like Dr. Crook had come to my home and said, *"Margaret, I'm going to write a book about you."*

After reading, marking and highlighting many pages of this book, I took it to my doctor and said, *"I know this is controversial, but the book sounds as though it was written about me. For one thing, it makes me feel my problems are yeast related because of the repeated courses of antibiotics I've taken for chronic urinary tract infections."*

My doctor said it was okay to go on a sugar-free diet, but he would not give me nystatin. He was concerned about side effects. So I went to a health food store and obtained some caprylic acid and I followed a sugar-free diet to the letter.

I then learned that a Chesapeake, Virginia, physician and his staff were interested in yeast-related illness. So I made an appointment. When I told the office nurse my story, she said, "Dr. Powell will be glad to talk to you," and she went to the bookshelf and brought me Dr. Crook's book, *Chronic Fatigue Syndrome and the Yeast Connection.* I could not believe it and I did not know that it existed. Dr. Powell and his staff were supportive and with their help I found that I was sensitive to a number of foods and food additives and preservatives.

During the next several years, I continued to improve and my symptoms gradually subsided. I also found that Dr.

Linda Rodriguez, a Virginia Beach physician, was interested in yeast problems. She recommended nutritional supplements and in a very short time I felt a lot better.

During the last five years I've continued to watch my diet and avoid chemicals and food additives, including MSG. I also continue the supplements every day. I now keep five-year-old twin grandchildren and an 18-month-old little brother. Also, my 89-year-old mother still lives with me.

I work with 12 teenagers in our church and serve as the director of a very active Puppet team. I'm chairman of our community National Day of Prayer every May and last, but not least, I'm now a member of the Advisory Board of Dr. Crook's International Health Foundation. I just wish I had more hours in the day to help educate more people, including the medical profession, about the "yeast connection" to many health problems.

◆◆◆ ⊠ ◆◆◆

Margaret and her husband, Louis, are wonderful friends. She came to Jackson to see me a couple of years ago and in the fall of 2000 she also came to Richmond to see me. She continues to do many, many things for me and for others.

Dr. Crook

Susan

D
ear Dr. Crook,
Dr. Geraldine Donaldson asked me to write you about my experience of being treated for candidiasis. I also received your letter, I don't know if you can use this, but feel free to use whatever meets the needs of your book. I believe my symptoms began about 22 years ago at the birth of my fifth child. I was 36 years old at the time and began to experience depression and fatigue and not feeling well. Everyone (myself included) thought I was just feeling overwhelmed with having 5 children in 9 years.

After a few years and worsening symptoms, I decided to see a doctor. I presented him with the following list of complaints: "I often feel like I'm coming down with the flu, but I don't actually get that sick. I feel achy, queasy, tired, scratchy throat, slightly sore glands on right side of my neck and feel depressed with little interest in doing much of anything. I also feel foggy brained a lot of the time."

He ran several lab tests all of which yielded normal results. At this point he recommended I see a psychologist. So off I went hopeful that this would be the answer to my problem. I worked with the psychologist for several months of talk therapy and antidepressants with only limited results. I did learn some important skills for emotional health, and unburdened myself of some important issues. However after about six months of treatment I was tested and found to be still clinically depressed. My therapist strongly felt that there was something physically wrong with me and sent me back to the doctor. He ran the tests again and again they came back normal. He advised me to go back to the therapist. I was starting to feel like a bouncing ball.

Over the next few years I did bounce back and forth between the doctor and the therapist and read every health related and self-help book I could find. It became the family joke. "We need to add on a room just to hold Mom's self help books."

In my searching I did come across a book that seemed to jump out at me at the book store. That book was, *The Yeast Connection,* by William G. Crook, M.D. This was about 12–15 years ago. As I read the symptoms and realized my personal history included long-term antibiotics, birth control pills (both as treatment for acne) and a diet heavy in sweets and carbohydrates, I felt that I had found the answer to my problem. I tried to treat myself with herbs and diet but ended up feeling worse.

At this point I knew I needed to have a doctor oversee the treatment. I found one who treated me with nystatin and low-carb diet. I came down with a bad case of the flu about 4 days into the treatment and afterward for three weeks I felt so weak I could hardly function. It wasn't a typical flu reaction for me. The weakness just wasn't going away so I went back to the doctor who told me that it was caused by the fact that my body wasn't using the protein for energy. He added carbohydrates and the weakness gradually went away and I gave up on this treatment for the time being. Now I know that this was caused by die-off. Appar-

ently this doctor was not very experienced with
ment and missed this point.

Ten years later I was still struggling. I had tried almost
every antidepressant made and many different kinds of supplements. One that did help some was blue green algae
(spirulina) which helped relieve the achiness and fatigue to
a degree. I had pretty much given up and decided that I
was just going to have to live with the symptoms . But fate
gave me another chance. Two years ago my daughter asked
me to attend a workshop on chronic fatigue she had signed
up for but was unable to attend. A discussion of candida
came up and the woman sitting next to me said she had
been successfully treated by a Dr. Geraldine Donaldson.

I decided to give the treatment another try and called
her the next day. This time the treatment was much more
complicated but proved to be effective and I did get a lot
of relief from my 20 year old symptoms. Dr. Donaldson's
treatment included the use of 2 antifungals, fluconazole and
miconazole.

She started me out gradually on each one so there was
no die-off reaction. The diet consisted of low carb vegetables
and meats. She had me tested for food allergies and found
I was allergic to several foods and molds. That required me
to follow rotation diet of foods I could eat as well as elimination of the allergic foods and yeast containing foods. I found
this very challenging at first. To succeed at this I knew I
would have to get creative and keep a positive attitude
because it was a lot of work.

In addition to the diet and medications I had to use a
sorbic acid nasal spray, Orithrush mouth wash, probiotics

twice a day and supplements; oil of primose, Vitamin C , B complex, multivitamins, calcium, flax seed oil, and douching with Citricidal.

After one month on the strict low-carb diet, I was allowed 50–60 carbs a day including fruit 3 times a week. This did not change for the rest of the treatment, I was not perfect however. There were definitely some bad days when I exceeded that by quite a bit, including sometimes dessert. I would get right back on the next day. There was one time when I didn't get back on and basically blew it for about 3 weeks. This was about 4 months into the treatment and I had to start back at square one.

But I went into it this time with a stronger commitment and was recovered 6 months later. Still I didn't always follow the plan perfectly. I still had those off days, but they were not very often. I believe part of the success came from my deciding to make it a game. Reading labels, trying new ways of preparing food, getting candida cookbooks. (My favorite recipe was the Creamy Spinach-Chicken Soup from the *Yeast Connection Cookbook*. I made double batches and froze it in individual soup bowls then popped them out and stored them in freezer bags.) Having food made ahead and handy made all the difference on those tired, feeling crummy days.

However the best source of help for me was prayer. I had strong emotional attachments to those sweet foods and on the bad days prayer got me through. Treating the allergies was another important part of the treatment. I hadn't realized how much I was affected by these foods. I was given antigen shots in addition to avoidance of certain foods. I was also treated with NAET (Nambudripad's Allergy Elimination Technique) by my chiropractor. This has helped with molds and specific foods. This treatment has given me back my life.

I feel blessed to have found an excellent doctor who really knew how to effectively treat this condition. I was able to go off my antidepressant about 3 months into the treatment and have felt no need for it since. I have more energy. I lost 35 lbs. My sore throat, achiness, queasiness, belching, flatulence, cough are gone. Even my nails got stronger.

Excluding sugar and white flour, I eat fairly normally now. I even have dessert occasionally. Although I don't enjoy them like I use to. I still have to avoid some things. (Too many vinegar products in one day makes me itchy.) All in all a tough program that is well worth the effort as it has formed new habits that brought me back to health. I was blessed to have found an excellent doctor whose treatment was very thorough and effective.

Susan Farr

◆◆◆ ◻ ◆◆◆

I met Dr. Donaldson at a conference of the American College of Environmental Medicine in the early 1990s. I also read the comprehensive instructions she gives her patients with yeast-related problems. I only wish there were thousands of physicians like Dr. Donaldson in the world to help polysymptomatic people who've been unable to find answers.

Dr. Crook

Thia

pril 10, 2000

Dear Dr. Crook:

It has been one year this month since I, by chance, found your book, *The Yeast Connection Handbook*, in a bookstore. I decided to take your advice, and it has changed my life in so many ways. I want to celebrate this one-year anniversary by writing to thank you. Seldom does one read a book that makes such an impact in ones life and lives up to so many of its promises.

My name is Thia. I am 50 years old, have one son, one stepson, and a husband, Steve. I teach seventh grade in a school system just outside Columbus, Ohio. I had seen an infomercial and was looking for the book it advertised in a bookstore when the phrase "sick all over" called to me from your book cover. The book was on the bottom shelf and I could not even see the title, but that phrase spoke volumes to me. I have felt "sick all over" for at least 12 years, and have dealt with other health issues most of my adult life.

I read the beginning, quickly took the little test to see if I qualified, and decided to buy the book. The next day was Saturday, and I did not get dressed until 2:00 in the afternoon because I could not stop reading your book. I was amazed. It spoke so clearly about so many problems I have dealt with. I decided that if I was not willing to try the suggestions, I could not complain any more about being sick.

It was not easy. As you predicted in the book, I felt worse the first two days and was "mad at the world." I would be hungry, and not be able to find anything to eat. Less than one week into it, I felt noticeably better, and it was all up hill from there. I spent several months in fear that my new found energy and well being would go away. I was sure this was just a "honeymoon period." This new sense of normalcy and health just could not last. But it did. It has never gone away. I am beginning to believe that it can last a lifetime.

I have changed the way I judge what I put into my body. I was overwhelmed at first, and for quite a while seemed to have more questions than answers. Now I still have more questions (daily), but know this is a lifelong process of learning. The information available changes constantly. It can still be difficult to know what is the best advice. I wrote to the nonprofit International Health Foundation in Tennessee for a list of physicians that support your program.

I now see Dr Sandra Pinkham in Columbus, Ohio. She has been very helpful. After seeing the change in me, people are constantly asking what I did. I now have 6 other friends who see her, and several others who have borrowed your book. I finally bought a second copy of *The Yeast Connection Handbook* so I could keep one to refer to. When people say to me, "I need to lose some weight. I want a copy of your diet," I just laugh. I tell them if they want to lose 20 lbs, go to Weight Watchers. When they hear the dietary changes I have made they often say they could never do that. I always tell them that if it made them feel as much better as it has made me feel, they could and would.

1988 is the year I remember as the beginning of feeling "bad all over." After years of doctors and testing and psychologists, chronic fatigue syndrome was the diagnosis given by one of them. I felt so sick sometimes I did not know anything to do but cry. When people would hear chronic fatigue, they would react by saying they knew how I felt because they got tired a lot too. The other common remark was that I did not look sick.

The name "Chronic Fatigue" did not describe the depth of the fatigue and its other symptoms. It felt like I had the flu. Even my skin would hurt. I constantly doubted my mental state. I had doctors ask me if my love life was satisfying, tell me I had heart problems and do cardio testing, and tell me to stay away from my dog. A psychologist was the first to suggest what was then called Epstein Barr virus. She gave me hope that there was a physical reason for my sickness. I sought counseling several times over the years to deal with depression.

I wanted to find the root of the prevailing sadness I often felt. I have been on some type of prescription medication constantly since my early 20s. I continued with my life and seldom missed work, but often wondered how I could make it through the day. I did get better, and would get sick less often, but it always returned. Each time I was surprised again at how sick I felt.

Another prevailing issue in my life has been compulsive eating. My weight has fluctuated between 150 and 200 lbs from my mid 20s on. I spent years attending Overeaters

Anonymous in search of help for my addiction to food. My success there was on and off also. That too I blamed on my weakness and lack of will power.

In the last few years I added vulvodynia to my list of discomforts. I did not have a history of yeast infections, but found myself unable to get rid of constant pain, burning and inflammation. I tried everything that was suggested to me by gynecologists, doctors, and friends, but Diflucan was the only thing that helped. But, that was not permanent. It would always start up again.

Today I can honestly say I have not felt depressed since I began this eating plan. Sad at times, yes, but not depressed. There is such a difference. I have lost about 50 lbs and my cravings for food are manageable and so much less obsessive. I am no longer on any prescription medication. I have not had a problem with chronic fatigue since last April. The vaginal inflammation is much improved. I started to exercise regularly last summer, and now on alternate days run about 1½ miles and do weight resistance and other exercises. I also take yoga classes.

My energy still amazes me (and my husband). I do not come home at the end of an exhausting day of teaching and hit the couch. I keep going until bedtime. My ability to sleep has changed too. I sleep better than I have in years and get up more easily in the morning. That is when I choose to exercise. Getting up in the morning used to be very hard for me. My husband teases me by saying our heating bill has dropped because I do not get as cold as I used to. My body temperature seems to have changed. I also noticed a difference this fall when I had 125 new names to learn. I felt that I remembered them more quickly and easily.

Life feels good and healthy and normal. Being sick in so many ways for so long really helps me appreciate that. Never a day goes by that I don't feel blessed by the changes in my life. Friends and coworkers comment often on the changes they notice: weight, skin color, eyes, and an overall sense that I am happier.

Currently, I try to be wheat, sugar, and dairy free. I eat few processed foods and watch my fat intake. I am enjoying experimenting with new foods and recipes. I take a good daily vitamin that contains most of your recommended vitamins and minerals. I use many of the food supplements you recommended also. Some eating situations are still difficult, but most of the time I find comfortable ways to take care of myself. The biggest overall difference in my life is that now I feel strong enough and care enough to work hard at taking care of myself—physically and mentally.

I have just started re-reading parts of *The Yeast Connection Handbook*. I already have a few things I want to try that I missed the first time through. I still have some relapses with vaginal burning, and sinusitis was a problem this winter. I see Dr Pinkham about every 6 months now and can e-mail her if needed.

This letter is to thank you for your part in changing my life and giving me back my health, I am sure you have heard many success stories, but I needed to share mine with you.

With gratitude,
Thia Thornburg

July 2001

I saw Dr. Pinkham today. I had my blood tests forwarded to her and I guess my family doctor misread my tests. His office called and told me my cortisol levels were normal so my adrenal glands were not the problem. Dr. Pinkham showed me that for one test—when I was feeling very bad—the morning level was 1.1 when the range went to 22. The bottom line is that my DHEA is low and my cortisol is very low at times and not consistent.

She says now that we have proof that it is an adrenal problem but not Addison's disease. I feel much better about everything thanks to the two of you. Patients really have to be on their toes today and be informed. Dr. Pinkham is adamant that I stay low stress and exercise moderately. Thanks again for your continued concern and support.

Sincerely,
Thia

August 2001 (E-mail)

I'm not back to normal, but I can tell that I'm healing and improving. I guess the adrenal problem will take some time to return to normal. I started some yoga most mornings and a little light weight lifting to try and resume getting some exercise. So far it has gone well. I feel much better about everything thanks to you and Dr. Pinkham.

During a long phone visit with Thia in August 2001 I told her of my strong interest in mild adrenal insufficiency and the re-

sponse of tired people with yeast-related problems to low dose cortisol therapy.

Dr. Crook

SECTION FOUR
Teens/ Children

Alyssa

A lyssa was born May 26, 1995. My labor had been induced with the drug pitocin. Initially everything seemed fine. But by 6 months we became concerned with Alyssa's development. She was making no attempts at babbling, was putting no weight on her legs and showed no signs of crawling. An unexplained vascular rash also appeared on her legs.

Alyssa had her first URI at 2 mos. and second at 4 mos., which included her first ear infection and first experience with antibiotics. This pattern continued until Alyssa was just about 2½ years old, had been prescribed antibiotic treatment 25 times, and had P.E. tubes surgically placed in her ears twice, at 9.5 mos. and 19 mos.

Alyssa began walking just as she turned 2, but her language was still severely delayed and she was evaluated as having sensory integration dysfunction. The rash still remained. We had seen many doctors and specialists about the strange rash, including a trip to the Mayo Clinic because of a possible but inconclusive diagnosis of a rare genetic disorder.

The summer after Alyssa's 2nd birthday, she began wheezing and developed pneumonia twice. This pattern continued, followed by a diagnosis of asthma and regular breathing treatments. Tubes were being recommended for a third time. We were frustrated and very worried. Traditional medical care was doing nothing to help our daughter. Alyssa's health was worsening and her delays were more pronounced.

It was when we began working with pediatrician Dr. Linda Rodriguez and pediatric allergist Dr. Richard Layton and read Dr. Crook's book *The Yeast Connection* that Alyssa's health began to change. Both doctors agreed, later confirmed by stool analysis, that Alyssa had a major overgrowth of candida, which contributed to a leaky gut, food allergies, and possibly her developmental delays and skin rash. They truly listened to our story and helped us take control of Alyssa's health by addressing the underlying issues.

Through nutritional intervention Alyssa's health improved almost immediately. To starve the candida yeast, Dr. Rodriguez had us eliminate all milk, white flour and refined sugar from Alyssa's diet. We also began an aggressive regime of Shaklee nutritional supplements to boost Alyssa's weakened immune system. Within a month we saw the most wonderful changes. Alyssa became more animated and smiled more (she felt better!), the asthma disappeared, the pattern of sickness which was once constant lessened greatly, and she was no longer on antibiotics!

Developmentally, Alyssa began making steady improvements. Alyssa just recently turned six. She has a very strong immune system, is actually healthier than the average child now, never has a need to be on antibiotics, and has made huge developmental gains. She will begin kindergarten in the fall. We have been very fortunate to have worked with wonderful practitioners, therapists, and teachers.

Alyssa has received both private and school based

speech, OT, and PT and in this last year craniosacral therapy as well. We have worked with Sandy Pranti, OT here in Cincinnati and have also had Alyssa treated at the Upledger Institute in FL.

We have watched Alyssa blossom before our eyes as a result of this therapy. But beyond a shadow of a doubt we know none of Alyssa's gains would have been possible without nutritional intervention, which we still continue regularly. That was our first and most important step in regaining Alyssa's health. We thank Dr. Rodriguez for sharing her wisdom and knowledge of healing with families like ours.

Alyssa's mother

•• •• •• ✉ •• •• ••

Dr. Rodriguez, a pediatrician, became interested in yeast-related disorders over a decade ago and she now serves as a valued member of the Advisory Board of the International Health Foundation.

Dr. Crook

John

At birth, in August 1985, John was a beautiful, healthy baby. Then he began to have colds and by the age of three months he developed repeated bouts of ear infections. These continued and by the age of four, he had received broad spectrum antibiotic drugs 15 times.

At 16 months, John developed a constant runny nose and two months later he became cranky and developed allergic shiners under his eyes. By age two he showed signs of hyperactivity, especially when he ate sweets. He didn't sleep and many nights he would be up five to ten times.

John was wild, constantly energetic, climbing on tables and counters. He even tried to climb out the kitchen window. He was accident prone and had to be stitched up several times. On one occasion it took 15 stitches to sew up his head. He was a real terror and would chase his family members with knives.

When John was four, I learned about yeast-related problems which people can develop by being given too many broad spectrum antibiotics. The antibiotics wipe out the good bacteria in the intestinal tract and candida yeasts overgrow and food particles seem to leak into the body, causing allergic reactions.

Through elimination diet and testing by an empathetic physician, we found that John was allergic to many different things, including foods and inhalants. Once treatment was started, which included a sugar free, yeast free diet, John improved dramatically. Yet, when he cheated on the diet his symptoms would come back.

WGC: In the late 1980s John's mother, Cathy, and I began to exchange letters and I met her for the first time in September 1997 at a conference in Tarrytown, NY. In late December 1998, she sent me a five page letter. Here are excerpts:

John was at one time a hyperactive child with behavior and learning problems. He is now a quiet (at times shy) calm, intelligent young man. Before he was treated for yeasts, he had problems with dyslexia. I kept copies of handwriting samples and he had problems sitting still long enough to focus on his work. He is a straight A student at the top of his class. He rarely studies because it seems that his memory works so well he doesn't need to. He goes to a private school, and although he is in the 8th grade, he is also taking 9th grade math.

John enjoys basketball, soccer and piano. He's even composed about 12 pieces of his own, some of which have been published. He's well liked by his classmates and friends. I continue John and his two siblings on a program which includes sugar-free vitamins, acidophilus, grape seed extract and calcium and magnesium supplements.

We follow the candida diet at home most of the time. Yet, the family goes off of it for parties and special occasions, but John doesn't seem to react adversely. None of us ever get sick and I use echinacea if anyone ever starts sneezing and that takes care of the problem within a day or two.

Overall, John is a pleasure to have as a son and we're all very proud of him. We wish you and your family a wonderful holiday season and a happy new year."

✦✦✦ ✉ ✦✦✦

In November 1999, Cathy told John's story at the Georgetown University conference, ADHD: Causes and Possible Solutions.

Dr. Crook

Douglas

In May 1999, I attended the conference in Orlando, Florida sponsored by Great Plains Lab. As I listened to Dr. Jeff Bradstreet, he made the comment that if you brought a child to him and that child had allergy problems, Dr. Bradstreet would send that child to Dr. Richard Layton in Maryland. So, my husband and I decided to have our family doctor run the preliminary tests that DAN! doctors required. We then made plans to go see Dr. Layton. Douglas has been in Dr. Layton's care for a year now.

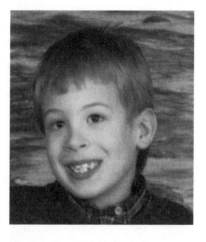

Douglas was allergic to everything Dr. Layton tested him for. Dr. Layton finds Douglas to be very tricky and extremely sensitive. Douglas now takes sublingual drops for food allergies. The best responses we have received during our treatment have been treatments to clean up and heal Douglas' gut! Since beginning treatment with Dr. Layton, Douglas went from over 50 ear infections at age 8 to only one in the last year!

Douglas takes a rice-based Florabiotic and Colostrom Gold which we obtained from Kirkman Labs and his response has been wonderful! His eyes are less dilated since the Colostrom. He learns better and his desire to socialize with other children skyrocketed.

Currently I would not call Douglas a "success" story—he is a "success" story in the making.

Kindest regards,
Christine Atkins

Jeff*

eff was born in June of 1985, and is now 16 years old. We learned soon after he was born that he had Down's Syndrome. To be honest, that diagnosis was very upsetting to us at first. However, Jeff did begin to develop and, by three months, he was smiling and responding to us. Unfortunately, he had very severe heart problems, and had to have heart surgery when he was three months old. During and following surgery, Jeff took lots of IV antibiotics. During the two days following surgery, Jeff had a very difficult time. His heart stopped beating eight different times. He was in intensive care for 14 days following surgery. When Jeff was finally released from the hospital, one of the nurses told us that he was the sickest child she had ever seen that had survived. All the other children she had seen that were as sick as Jeff had died.

When Jeff came home from the hospital, he was 4 months old and weighed only seven pounds. During his first winter, he got sick three times. Each time he had to go back to the hospital. The first time he had pneumonia, for which he had IV antibiotics. We knew that antibiotics would cause yeast problems, but it seemed that there was no choice. One

---

*Jeff's mother, Kathy Gibbons, Ph.D., received her degree in biochemistry from the University of Illinois. You can send a message to her at Healthy Actions,5300 DTC Parkway, #210, Greenwood Village, CO 80111 or healthyactions@aol.com.

week after the first illness, Jeff was back in the hospital with a different kind of pneumonia that he had caught from being in the hospital the first time. This second illness meant more IV antibiotics. Then another week later he had a third illness, which was picked up during his second hospital stay. That third illness led to another hospital stay and more IV antibiotics. Finally we took him home.

At ten months Jeff began to feel a little better and have some energy. At that time we thought that he was stable enough to tolerate a treatment for yeast. We really wanted to treat the yeast because he had had so many antibiotics before he was even one year old. Diflucan was not available then, but nystatin was. We gave him powdered nystatin prescribed by Dr. Del Stigler, Jeff's pediatrician. We also tried many over-the-counter yeast treatments. The combined effect was that Jeff began to grow and thrive.

When Jeff was two years old we took him to see Dr. Sidney Baker, who helped us a great deal with many different aspects of Jeff's health. When Jeff was four years old, Dr. Baker called and said that he knew about a new drug that he thought might help Jeff. It was available only from England, and was called Diflucan. We started him on 50 mg per week, and it was very effective. For the first time Jeff was able to sit down on the couch and pay attention when we read a book to him. Diflucan made a tremendous improvement in Jeff's attention span within 24 hours of the first dose.

When he was four, we began to give him growth hormone. A conventional overnight test for growth hormone had indicated that Jeff had no detectable amount of that hormone. Our pediatric endocrinologist prescribed one shot each evening of growth hormone, which improved Jeff's muscle tone enormously. At that same time, Jeff began to take Piracetam, which was prescribed by Dr. Baker. Piracetam definitely improved Jeff's articulation.

When Jeff reached the age to enter school, we became very upset with the public school system because it seemed that the administrators had a stereotype of what a Down's Syndrome child should be able to do and were not willing to evaluate Jeff's particular situation. We sent him to a regular private preschool, which was very good because Jeff got lots of good modeling from the other children. We had a videotape made of him at the preschool interacting with the other children. We gave the tape to the principal of the local public elementary school, and, after reviewing the tape, the principal agreed to accept Jeff as a student at that school.

During the summer before Jeff was to enter kindergarten, we felt that he was ready to go in all ways except that he was not toilet trained. Dr. Del Stigler, as well as Dr. Baker, thought that Jeff was not toilet trained because he had an irritable bladder arising from food allergies. An Immuno Labs food allergy test was done, and we found that wheat was a major problem. We removed wheat from Jeff's diet, and he was toilet trained within 24 hours. It seems that wheat was irritating his bladder, so he had to go to the bathroom very frequently. When wheat was taken out of Jeff's diet, he could go three hours between bathroom visits.

The allergy test also indicated that eggs were a problem. We did a classic elimination test by removing eggs from Jeff's diet for five days, and then put eggs back in on the sixth day. The most unbelievable thing happened. We remember so clearly that day. It was an afternoon in June, and we were sitting outside at our picnic table. We gave Jeff some egg salad, and within 20 minutes he was stuttering so badly that he could hardly get a single word out. We were very impressed that the Immuno Labs test picked up both the egg and the wheat allergies.

When Jeff was in the first grade, he did EPD treatments with Dr. Shrader in Santa Fe, NM. That treatment improved Jeff's focus. Jeff had been labeled by several teachers as an ADD or ADHD child. When Jeff has had lots of food he is allergic to, then he acts like he has ADD or ADHD. But when he sticks to his diet and avoids foods he is allergic to, then he doesn't behave like an ADD or ADHD child at all. When he follows the diet, he is very focused, and he behaves very well.

When Jeff was in the second grade we treated him with a month of Diflucan. That treatment was extremely helpful at improving his performance in school. His attention span was much improved following that treatment. When Jeff was in the fourth grade, we treated him with a month of Lamisil. We decided to try it because his toenails looked like the pictures of fungal toenails that all the drug company representatives were handing out. His toenails got much better. But, even more importantly, his behavior and concentration improved.

Jeff attended kindergarten through fifth grade in a regular public elementary school in an integrated program in a normal classroom. The other children were very accepting of him. He learned to read at the third grade level. He is much better at grasping concrete ideas rather than abstract thinking. We moved to a new school district during the summer before Jeff started sixth grade. We wanted Jeff to be able to continue in an integrated program, and the old district would not provide that option. In the new district he attended integrated classrooms in social studies and science.

I am totally convinced that yeast is a big part of the picture for Jeff. When his yeast is high, he does not concentrate and his behavior is very scattered. All of the antifungal treatments that we have given him have been very helpful.

So now Jeff is off to high school starting in the fall of 2001. He is scheduled to take a reading class. He reads *Sports Illustrated* on his own and enjoys it. Jeff will also be taking some job training. Jeff will be focusing on classes that prepare him for what he will be doing after high school. Jeff turned 16 just 2 months ago. He is 5 feet and 5 inches tall, which is a reasonable height for a Down's Syndrome child. We think that the growth hormone helped him grow and also improved his muscle tone. Maybe the improved muscle tone carried over to improved muscle tone in his heart muscle. That would be nice if it happened because Jeff still has a weak mitral valve, even though his heart surgery was eventually successful.

Jeff stopped growth hormone about one year ago. It seemed that he did not need that boost any longer. He had grown well and his muscle tone was good. He has continued to grow well for a year without the growth hormone and his muscle tone has continued to be good.

✦✦✦ ✉ ✦✦✦

I met Kathy, a professional with impeccable academic and personal credentials in Denver in the mid 1990s. Since that time we've become friends and I've sought her help and consultation on a number of occasions. In July 2000 I called her to obtain information about electroacupuncture testing and diagnosis, and with her permission I recorded our conversation. I included excerpts of our conversation in my 2001 book, **Tired—So Tired! and the "yeast connection."**

As Paul Harvey would say, "Here's the rest of the story." In June 2001 I went to Colorado for Kathy to carry out electroacupuncture testing on me. Her findings have helped me tremendously.

Dr. Crook

Kristie

When our six-year-old daughter, Kristie, was almost three years old, she began having ear infections—one right after the other. During the next year, she developed such severe behavior problems that our pediatrician sent us to a children's hospital and to a child-development center in Louisville. They said Kristie was very bright and when they couldn't find anything wrong, they said, "She has a behavior problem." None of their suggestions helped.

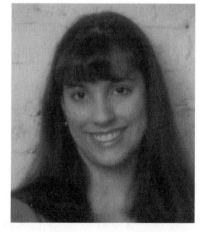

Our pediatrician then sent us to Dr. J. T. Jabbour at LeBonheur Children's Hospital in Memphis. Dr. Jabbour tried different drugs but none of them helped. Then he said, *"Her behavior could be caused by something she's eating."*

In March of 1989, we put Kristie on an elimination diet. On adding foods back, we found that chocolate, sugar, food dyes, yeast and wheat triggered her nervous system symptoms. Then we brought her to you, and because she had so many ear infections, you prescribed nystatin. You also recommended vitamins, magnesium, flaxoil and other supplements. We also took her off packaged foods containing sugar and dyes and fed her well-balanced meals.

Today our little girl is a changed person. She smiles, giggles and laughs. She's no longer "klutzy" like she was before. Her sleeping patterns have drastically improved. She's agreeable and her behavior has totally changed. She's doing well in kindergarten and her teachers can't believe she was ever hyperactive.

The diet and treatment program is so simple I can't believe doctors won't at least try elimination diets first, rather than automatically putting children on drugs. This program has changed Kristie's life and ours, too.

Cheryl and Stanley Loe

I saw Kristie many times during the early and mid-1990s and her mother was diligent in carrying out a comprehensive treatment program. Although Kristie experienced occasional problems because she reacted adversely to several different chemicals, she continued to improve each year. Major credit for her improvement belongs to her parents who conscientiously and consistently carried out the recommended treatment program.

Because I hadn't seen Kristie in several years, I called her mother in May 2001. Here are excerpts from our conversation.

Kristie's doing great in school. She is a senior in high school and if she maintains her current grade point average, she will graduate as an honor graduate. She's taking her ACT test and she's going to see about volunteering at the hospital this summer. She's decided she wants to be a nurse. She's going to start out at the community college in Paducah where they have a two-year nursing program. After that she's not sure. She wants to work in the nursery with the babies. Her health is fine and she was absent only a couple of days from school this past year.

I know that Kristie taking the nystatin definitely helped her, but she hasn't taken it for many years. With her health being better, she hasn't had as many antibiotics. When we decided about her chemical allergies, I think this was a very big step toward her improvement. After switching from gas to an all-electric house, we saw changes almost daily.

She still takes nutritional supplements and allergy drops for inhalants, chemicals and foods, along with the antihistamine Zyrtec. She used to couldn't tolerate chocolate, but she can now. She knows not to go overboard and she eats just about anything. She eats well-balanced meals including fruits and vegetables. She is 5'4" and weighs 115.

Kristie has grown into a beautiful young woman and we are so very proud of her many accomplishments.

◆ ◆◆ ◆◆ ⊠ ◆◆ ◆◆ ◆

Like every person whose success story I've included in this book, Kristie's improvement is due to many, many things—especially attention to and control of diet and limitation to exposure to environmental chemicals.

Dr. Crook

Sam

lmost a decade ago, I established **Parents of Allergic Children** and began working to help parents and children with behavior and learning problems. Here's what motivated me.

My youngest son, Sam (not his name), now 17 years old, was one of these complicated kids and had been diagnosed "developmentally delayed." I saw Dr. Rapp on the Phil Donahue show in 1988, called her office and went to one of her colleagues in New York. This doctor put Sam on a diet and although he improved a lot, he continued to have problems.

Then we went to Dr. Alan Lieberman, a South Carolina pediatrician, who checked Sam for candida. Dr. L. prescribed four days of Nizoral and then nystatin for three months. Since that time Sam hasn't been troubled with yeast-problems.

In the first grade Sam's teacher told me that he was experiencing trouble learning to read and wasn't paying attention. She implied that he had ADD and I didn't want to put him on Ritalin and other drugs. Then, I found out about an allergy blood test, the ELISA test, which helped identify dietary ingredients that were causing problems. Sam took this test and we learned that he was sensitive to gluten and many other things

Within a week after changing his diet and eliminating these foods, he could read a chapter in a book without difficulty. All of his grades went up and his learning disability and attention symptoms went away.

When people in my community started seeing that I knew something, they'd tell others to talk to me. Other parents have used tests which came from Great Smokies Lab, Metrametrix Lab and have found answers.

Sam is doing great now. He will be a senior this year. Last year he was on the honor roll and took some honor courses. He got a good score on his SAT test. His low muscle tone has gone away and he's now a black belt in Taekwondo. He won the most improved swimmer on the swim team a couple of years ago. He is an Eagle Scout and wants to be a meteorologist.

Many things that we did played an important part in helping him, including antiyeast medications, avoiding sugar, dairy and gluten-containing foods and other foods that caused sensitivity reactions. Vitamins and antioxidants were also important parts of Sam's treatment program. In fact, my husband and I always say that Co-Enzyme Q_{10} is what cured his muscle problems. Dr. Lieberman worked with us and helped Sam with these therapies.

When Sam was in the 5th grade he started taking digestive enzymes. Before we made all the changes Sam was tired all the time and wanted to sleep. He now enjoys going out with his friends and rides his bicycle every day. He doesn't want to feel that way again, so he doesn't eat foods that disagree with him.

Because most physicians still don't know about food allergies and yeast-connected health problems, I now reach people through **Parents of Allergic Children.***

❧❧❧ ✉ ❧❧❧

In the early 1990s I first learned about the work of Parents of Allergic Children and I was impressed by the dedicated, unselfish work the members of this organization were doing to help children and their parents. I became even more impressed when I participated in a conference sponsored by Parents of Allergic Children in 2000.

Dr. Crook

*P.O. Box 1808, Midlothian, VA 22113, www.parentsofallergicchildren.org

Rachel

I n October 1992 I received the following letter from Rachel's mother, Kathleen.

Dear Dr. Crook:

My daughter Rachel started having headaches and stomach aches after a bout with the flu in December 1986. She had the urge to urinate all the time and complained of being tired. She developed asthma, and would get bronchitis every October. The doctors treated her with numerous antibiotics and medications. She gradually became worse and worse. We took her to numerous specialists—no doctor could find a medical reason for all her complaints.

From 1989 to 1990 she missed 97 days of school. She would lay on the couch all day and dunk her head in a bowl of ice water for relief from her headaches. She was so weak, the doctors suggested we take her to Diamond Headache Clinic. I made an appointment with them—but luckily I saw a doctor on T.V. talking about *The Yeast Connection*.

She would always tell the doctors that she felt "sick all over." I ran out and bought the book and stayed up until 4:00 A.M. reading it. It seemed as if it was written about Rachel. The next morning I called her neurologist and pediatrician and asked them about it. The neurologist said it could be part of her problem. The other doctor never heard of it and didn't believe a young child would suffer from chronic yeast infection.

We went to see the kind, knowledgeable, wonderful Chicago physician, Dr. George Shambaugh—and the rest is history. Thank you Dr. Crook from the bottom of our hearts. I continue to sing your praises.

Kathleen and Rachel Pawelczyk

After reading her letter, I wrote to Kathleen and sent her a questionnaire which I asked her to fill out and return to me. Here was one of my questions: **What treatment measures were most important in helping Rachel regain her health?** *(List them numerically, with #1 being most important.)*

In her reply, Kathleen put a #1 after each one of the options I listed.

⋄ *Antiyeast medications*
⋄ *Sugar-free special diet*
⋄ *Avoidance of food allergens*
⋄ *Avoidance of environmental pollutants*
⋄ *Allergy vaccines*
⋄ *Nutritional supplements*

She also circled Diflucan and made the following comments: "My daughter needed all the treatment measures above equally—if we varied from any of them she would start to become ill again. After a year and a half of treatment she has been able to switch to nystatin, may have sugar once in a while and is attending school full time this year. She's 98% improved since beginning treatment."

To get an update on Rachel I called Kathleen in April 2001. Here's an excerpt of what she had to say.

Rachel is now in New York. She still gets headaches at times, but she's not following the program as closely as she should. Periodically she'll go back on the acidophilus and everything to help with the yeast overgrowth. She said she knew she felt best when she was on the nystatin. She knows herself when she starts getting a headache because she's not on the program like she was before. She was going to the College of Dramatic Art but she took off this semester and she's now working as an assistant at HBO.

Tabitha

I n February 2001 I received a number of e-mail messages from Kathy Vernier of Stuarts Draft, Virginia. In her messages Kathy told me about her daughter's long struggle with respiratory problems. Here are excerpts.

Tabitha had been troubled by sinus problems, bronchitis and recurrent bouts of asthma since early childhood. Because of these problems she's taken many antibiotics and other medications. She's also been hospitalized several times. Then, three years ago, we took her to Dr. George Ward, a physician in the Allergy Department of the University of Virginia.

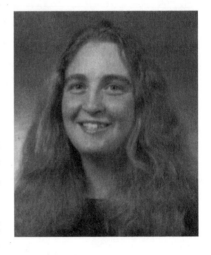

As you know, he was the senior author of the 1999 article published in a major allergy journal document- ing his success in treating patients with skin fungal in- fections and asthma using Diflucan. Although Tabitha gave no history of skin fungal infections, he prescribed Diflucan and it has proved to be a wonder drug in enabling her to overcome her asthma and lead a normal life.

To get more information I called Tabitha in May 2001 and with her permission I recorded our conversation. Here are excerpts of a typescript of our conversation.

It seems like I'd have bronchitis two or three times a year. It would start with a bad cough and runny nose and it would turn into bronchitis. It would be treated with some sort of antibiotic. That would take care of the infection, but the cough would stay.

I'd end up with a cough that would keep me up all night and keep my family up. It just wouldn't go away. They tried all sorts of drugs on me. That's how I ended up at UVa for allergy tests. The only test I showed positive to was dust mites. Then I was given Diflucan and within a week the cough was gone and I'd had it for about three months.

My family doctors continued to give me Diflucan, two or three times a week. I can't say I'm perfect in doing that, but whenever I feel an infection coming on I up the dose and take it for a couple of days and the cough clears up. That's pretty much where I am right now. I haven't had bronchitis for a while. I think I had one little flare up a couple of months ago. It got taken care of with an antibiotic and Diflucan.

In the past I would wheeze when I coughed and the Albuterol inhaler seemed to work best. The doctors also gave me the inhaled steroids and they didn't help. I used one for a few weeks and it never made any real difference. I'm really doing well. The only thing that causes me to cough now is when I'm around cigarette or wood smoke.

As long as I'm careful I stay in good shape. I've finished

my first year in college and right now I'm working on a farm as an animal caretaker with dogs. I also belong to a gym and my friends and I go there. I can run a good distance.

WGC: Do you remember how much time you missed when you were a freshman and sophomore in high school?

I missed a week and a half because of a cough. I couldn't get any sleep at night and it got to the point where they asked me to stay home because the other students couldn't hear the teacher when I was coughing. The problem wasn't any worse in the winter than it was in the summer. It didn't seem like there was a rhyme or reason to it when I started getting sick.

The doctors gave me a lot of antibiotics for my bronchial and sinus infections and I was almost never clear of sinus infections. I guess I grew accustomed to them. I have almost no sinus congestion or stuffy nose now. Although the doctors found I was allergic to dust and I got the hypoallergenic stuff (which seemed to help), nothing really helped until I began the Diflucan treatment two and a half years ago.

Wesley

hree-year-old Wesley was referred to me in August 1982 for evaluation of hyperactivity, irritability, peevishness and behavior problems. His mother said, "This child is driving me up the wall. I don't know how much longer his father and I can take it. He doesn't sleep, he's always on the go, he tears up his toys and wears out the furniture."

In reviewing Wesley's history I found that at the age of two months he was troubled by a persistent yeast infection in his mouth and diaper area. A month later, he developed an ear infection which was treated with a ten-day course of antibiotics. At four months, he was treated for another ear infection and the yeast infections in his mouth and diaper area flared up.

During the next year, Wesley had repeated—almost continuous—ear infections. Because of these problems he was given ampicillin, amoxicillin, Ceclor and other broad spectrum antibiotics. Between the ages of 18 and 24 months he became unusually aggressive, irritable and hard to manage. Symptoms were triggered by exposure to colognes, after shave lotions, perfumes and other odors.

Between the ages of two and two-and-a-half his nervous symptoms continued and included poor sleep and long-lasting temper tantrums. His symptoms were so severe the family was referred to a clinical psychologist for consultation. The psychologist told the parents to give Wesley more attention when he behaved well and to ignore his bad behavior. Those techniques didn't help and Wesley's nervous symptoms continued.

Because of his history of repeated antibiotics, I prescribed a yeast-free, sugar-free diet, nystatin and nutritional supplements. During a visit a week later Wesley's mother reported, "He's like an entirely different child. When he eats sugar or yeast-containing foods, his symptoms return."

At a followup visit on May 1, 1983, Wesley's mother commented,

Wesley's on nystatin and diet and he's doing great. We had only one outbreak of hyperactivity . . . this past Sunday . . . at a wedding celebration. He ate a piece of wedding cake and drank two cups of punch. That night he was in terrible shape. He's doing so much better and he now sits down and looks at books. He can be taken places without tearing the place apart. He's very cooperative and things are running smoothly.

In follow up reports in November 1983, November 1984 and July 1985, Wesley's mother reported that following the diet and taking nystatin are necessary to keep him out of trouble. Here's an excerpt from a letter Wesley's mother sent me in 1987.

He's finishing the second grade and is doing well. No problems with behavior and learning as long as he continues his treatment program which includes the special diet and small doses of nystatin. Corn and sugar seem to especially cause problems.

In the fall of 1993, I called Wesley's mother to find out how he was getting along. She told me he was doing fine and she wrote me a letter to put in his chart. Here are excerpts.

My son Wesley had repeated ear infections and took many, many antibiotics. We never spent a day that he hadn't cried. He never slept the whole night through. His outbursts were such that we were afraid he was going to hurt himself or someone in the family.

When we took him to a physician we were told to send him to a mental health doctor. Yet, we found on our own that sugar made a big difference. Then after our visit with you we put him on a low sugar diet, nystatin, magnesium and vitamins. The results were amazing. Within a three to four week period a different child emerged.

We now had a calm easy going child who was actually sitting on the floor, feet in the front, looking at the book. We had to take his picture because we had never seen him slow down enough to do this before.

Wesley is now 14 years old and he still follows a good diet and takes a good supply of vitamins, magnesium and nystatin to control yeast in his body. He never had to take Ritalin or other drugs. He's doing well in self-esteem and in his school work.

I have followed Wesley over the years. Wesley's mother has called me and sent me letters and reports over the years and in March 2000 she said,

He graduated from high school and has held a responsible job for the past three years. On April 15th he'll be married.

SECTION FIVE
Men

Bob

1

982–1983

My patient suffered severe headaches every month, often requiring narcotics and bed rest. Attempts at dietary manipulation with little effect. His wife admitted to me at church one Sunday that she had taken him to see John Curlin two weeks earlier.

"How is he?," I asked.

She replied, "I have not been living for 30 years with the man I've been living with the last two weeks. He's been grouchy, irritable and impossible to please."

Bob heard the statement and said, "Paul, I want to defend myself. I've felt bad and had a continuous headache since I started the nystatin and got off all the sugar and yeast. Just in the last 1 or 2 days I seem to be getting better."

Eleven months later my wife and I met Bob and his wife for dinner at a local restaurant. Bob was careful to quiz the waiter about how things were prepared before he would order. While waiting on the meal, I asked, "How are the headaches?"

Bob said, "I have had **one**—I didn't know the sauce was made with mushroom gravy."

For the past 13 years Bob has continued to take nystatin daily and avoid desserts and obvious "fungus" foods and too much bread. He reports about one headache a year—whenever he inadvertently eats something he knows not to.

No toxicity to long term nystatin use seen.

PS—Bob is a professional licensed exterminator. He has worked in food handling plants as sanitation/compliance inspector for years. His wife is a retired school teacher. They are both highly educated and degreed.

Paul Schwartz, M.D.

Demetrius*

I'm fifty years old and have suffered for more than twenty years from all of the maladies so vividly described in your yeast connection books. I was sufficiently impressed with the advice in your book that I talked my doctor into giving me a prescription for nystatin. Amazingly, within a few hours, I felt a substantial improvement in my overall condition and now after a few weeks of treatment—

1. I don't suffer from general feelings of fatigue and malaise.
2. My stomach (which had been diagnosed as "nervous," "pre-ulcerated" or "hiatal hernia") immediately settled down.
3. I found my general state of well being improved dramatically.

Also, within a few days, my athlete's foot and jock itch, which had been part of my life for years, began to clear up.

I would be glad to provide more accurate and valuable information to a researcher who would like to talk to me and would be happy to make this information available to you and your team for analysis.

---

*Not his real name.

Let me extend my thanks to Dr. Truss for his scientific research and to you for making this information known to me and to many others. I don't really understand what the hell is going on, but I'm glad to feel normal for the first time in many years.

Ed

D r. Crook,

I believe that you "saved" another person's life with the knowledge I obtained from your book. I want to thank you for this. Your book was recommended to me through a friend that has a lot of knowledge in your field. I would be happy to share more details with you by phone or e-mail but I want to give you the basic details here just in case you want to document this.

More than a dozen mental health professionals in the business failed to catch the correlation of my brother's mental health state and his outward physical symptoms of fungus during the past twelve months, even after I repeatedly attempted to get them to focus on this having copied your article for each of them.

My brother, 46 years old, came to us in April 2000 having been addicted to pain killers for the past 20–25 years, indicating he could no longer take care of himself. He went through detox, had terrible diarrhea for 3 months and physically could not get off a couch. He had a toe nail fungus so bad that his toenails were totally destroyed. He has had this over ten years.

He had fungus in his groin area and buttocks that looked like acid burns. He was totally depressed, fatigued, talked of death all the time. He had OCD symptoms and was repetitive in his speech which was totally negative. He was helpless. He was first diagnosed with Aspergers Disorder, dual diagnosis, the schizophrenia and depression with psychotic features; all from different mental health doctors.

He attended day therapy classes which did no good whatsoever. He refused to take any medication such as Prozac. He was cheeking the capsules and then we found out he emptied all the capsules and put the empties back in the container. We could not understand why there was no improvement until we discovered this. He ended up within 6 months, somewhat suicidal and psychotic and was involuntarily committed to Georgia Regional Hospital for 3 months.

He was given Haldol which was devastating to him. It turned him into a zombie and created Parkinson-like symptoms. There was no improvement with or without the Haldol. This was only administered for a couple of weeks. I finally convinced the doctor, after two months, to give him the Lamisil which had been recommended three times during this ordeal by three different doctors but only at our insistence did they finally agree to try this. (Unknown to us, at the time, how expensive this was.)

However, they wanted to treat his mental problems first and not complicate it with another medication. The doctor at Georgia Regional told me she was aware of anti-fungal treatments on patients with Ed's problem but did not do anything about it.

After four weeks on Lamisil, there was an amazing difference, much to our amazement. He started to look for a job, started driving, working out and conversing in a positive normal manner. He admitted that he did not take any of the medications at Georgia Regional (was faking it, cheeking, throwing away) despite our warnings to them that we knew he was doing this. We warned them to keep a close watch and they started to put the pills in powder form to drink. I don't know how he got away with it, supposedly being watched very closely.

He refused taking these drugs because he thought it made him more fatigued and could hardly get out of bed each day. He did not shower for a month until he was finally forced to do so.

The doctor at Georgia Regional made him sign a form saying that the Lamisil was not being given to him to treat his mental health symptoms and that the possibility of death from taking this anti-fungal drug existed.

He was attending a program called Vistas (day program) which is sponsored by the Northside Mental Health Division in North Atlanta, three days a week. He kept telling us everyone there was spaced out and walked around like zombies. He was supposed to have been on Prozac and Seraquil (but not taking it). He did not want to end up looking like them.

No matter who I spoke to, they did not believe me that I thought it might be the fungus he's had for so many years that was affecting him.

When Ed was in his 20's he took antibiotics for severe acne and boils and staph infections. He was always lazy, unmotivated, fatigued (but finally realized this fungus may be the cause of the problem). When he was prescribed this antifungal medication about ten years ago, he refused to take it as he was told it would take about a year to clear up this toenail fungus. He has already had two toenails removed.

I took an aggressive and active position on getting treatment for my brother. Many mental health doctors and counselors failed us along the way. He was an extreme case which caused everyone in our family terrible anguish and pain. All the procedures he had to go through to get to this point could have been aborted with taking Lamisil. He even had a colonoscopy for the diarrhea and found no infection except a slight irritation in the stomach and intestines. Our thought was cancer but fortunately it was not.

He was so far removed from reality we could not reason with him to take Lamisil initially. He did not think anything was going to work and he was going to die anyway.

At the writing of this fax to you which was January of 2001, he had been on the Lamisil for 4 weeks. He has had blood work done to check the liver to make sure it was not being affected.

You suggested Diflucan which would give the same results but not quite as harsh on the system and would eliminate the blood work. He now has been on Diflucan for perhaps four or five months now and takes the prescribed dosage one time a week.

Now he is a totally different person. Drives, cuts the lawn, goes to concerts, interested in TV and sports.

Carol

Enrico

By the grace of God and the help of a Dallas nutritionist and pharmacist, I was led to your book. I would have been in terrible shape if it had not been for the help of these two caring people.

For two and a half years, I had been saturated with eczema which covered my entire body and the itching was almost unbearable. I slept only about two to four hours nightly. Nothing I did, including consultation with five well-meaning doctors, seemed to help.

In July, I started taking nystatin and following the diet. I gradually began to improve. By September, I began to notice a real change. Now, three months after starting treatment, my body is clear and I'm sleeping most of the night without itching.

I'm beginning to feel like new again and I'm wondering how in the world I survived the last two and a half years. Thank you for caring enough to write your books. Please keep it up. My prayers are that anyone who needs to know about candida will make the discovery given to me.

Tom*

orty-one-year-old Tom's† chief complaints were asthma for four years, rectal itching, weight loss and secondary stress. His medical history included increased tonsillitis from ages 8–15 and the use of tetracycline for teenage acne. The need for antibiotics was minimal from approximately 1980–1998.

Tom's allergies including increased nasal symptoms which had begun about age five, and improved when he limited dairy products in 1995. However, he continued to have a persistent mild stuffiness and post nasal drip.

When Tom first came to see me his major concern was asthma which he first noted during his early 30s while exercising. Then the symptoms became more frequent and were also triggered by respiratory infections and increased coughing. He said his symptoms were worse in the middle of the night, and when swallowing. His complaints included tightness, shortness of breath and wheezing.

The bronchial inhaler, Albuterol, 1 puff twice daily helped relieve his symptoms. High doses caused adverse side effects. The steroid inhaler, Aerobid, 1 puff twice daily also helped. His asthma was better outside of the house compared to inside.

---

*Not his real name.

†Richard M. Layton, M.D., Towson, MD, sent me this story of Tom Johnson (not his name), a patient he saw for the first time in December 1998.

His other major complaints were rectal itching, bleeding and scabbing. An important point that he made was **with increased asthma, there was decreased rectal itching and vice versa.** And an inhaled steroid triggered his rectal itching, but helped his asthma.

Tom was also concerned by his 20 lb weight loss during the three years before his first office visit. He had been avoiding wheat, tomato and soy for two months and he avoided milk for six months before his first visit. He'd also received allergy testing at Johns Hopkins Hospital and was found to be negative for pollens, dust mold and dog. Foods were not tested.

In discussing his problems with him I said, "Tom, I think you have a yeast problem and in all likelihood, a food/leaky gut plays a part in causing your complaints."

Physical examination was within normal limits except for mold allergic shiners, an allergic appearance to the turbinates in his nose and severe perianal fungal dermatitis. This was treated with topical antifungal Loprox cream.

He was also tested for dust products, molds and foods. A yeast culture showed the rhodoturula yeast that was very sensitive to Nizoral and mildly sensitive to nystatin, caprylic acid and garlic. I started Tom on a probiotic, followed by "yeast fighters" two weeks later, and then a 10-day course of Nizoral, which caused increased fatigue.

At a follow-up visit two months later (February 1999) Tom was better. The Loprox ointment had helped his rectal itching and his treatment program included food and inhalant immuno-therapy, probiotics and "yeast fighters." Following this treatment program had helped Tom control both his asthma and his rectal itching.

I recommended another two-week course of Nizoral, 200 mg daily, to further control his yeast problem. Then during his visit in April 1999, Tom reported he continued to do well on 100 mg of Nizoral. Then I changed his treatment program to Diflucan 100 mg daily for one week, followed by 200 mg daily. He said, "I feel a lot better, think more clearly and all in all I'm feeling great."

At his next follow up visit (December 1999), Tom had been given Keflex for an infected bite. He had been continued on the Diflucan 200 mgs daily for two months, then decreasing to 100 mgs per day, he reported he was able to start running and lift weights for the first time in a year. He also used the inhaled steroids Pulmicort and Albuterol, 1 puff of each daily, to control his asthma.

In his last visit (June 2000), he said he was enjoying his best health in years. He continued to take Diflucan, which had been tapered down to 50 mg three times a week. When he tried to cut the dose down further his asthma worsened. On this dose his asthma, sleep, fatigue and rectal itching all improved. He was able to stop immunotherapy on this visit, although he continued to avoid foods he was allergic to, take probiotics and the Pulmicort and Albuterol when needed.

To summarize, Tom had both allergic asthma and a yeast problem. With the use of even low-dose steroid inhalers to control his asthma, his yeast problem flared up. On a good diet, appropriate supplements, antifungal medication, immunotherapy for one and a half years, he's enjoyed excellent health.

SECTION SIX

Comments
of
Physicians

Sidney M. Baker, M.D.

During *the past two decades, Dr. Baker, a former member of Yale University's School of Medicine, has said repeatedly,* "Labeling diseases isn't the way we should go." *Here are examples of what he and other physicians have said on this subject.*

When a person is tired and suffers from other chronic complaints, it's important for the physician to ask these two questions:

⋄ Is there something that this person needs that she is lacking?
⋄ Is there something that she is getting too much of that contributes to her problem?

Together, these two questions form the basis for detective work aimed at uncovering imbalances in people of all ages, with various problems. Essential lacks include:

⋄ nutrients provided by a good diet, including essential fatty acids, magnesium, B vitamins, zinc and other trace minerals.
⋄ full spectrum light

◇ clean air
◇ pure water
◇ love, praise, touch and other psychological nutrients
◇ exercise

The things a person should avoid as much as possible are:

◇ pollutants in the air, food, soil and water (such as pesticides, tobacco smoke and odorous chemicals)
◇ nutritionally poor foods and beverages (such as those which have been processed, packaged and loaded with sugars or containing coloring, additives and bad fats)
◇ allergens
◇ harmful microorganisms (including yeasts and other fungi, bacteria, viruses and parasites).

Even before Dr. Baker made his classic comments, Emanuel Cheraskin, M.D., D.M.D., a faculty member of the University of Alabama, in an article, "The Name of the Game is the Name," said in effect,

We physicians are taught to diagnose, classify and label diseases. And most of us feel if we can put a diagnostic label on each patient who comes to us we've done our duty. Then we can relax because our task becomes easy.

All we have to do then is go to our procedure book, medical library, Physician's Desk Reference (PDR) or computer and find the recommended treatment. Then we prescribe drugs, surgery or psychotherapy.

*And in his pioneer book **Predictive Medicine,** Cheraskin said that many disabling disorders could be prevented by recognizing early signs and symptoms. He emphasized that patients with many of these disorders could be helped when they change their diets and their lifestyles.*

*In his book, **The Missing Diagnosis,** Dr. Orian Truss commented,*

I would like to call attention once again to the pitfall inherent in dividing human illness into "diseases." The organs and systems of the body are so integrated, with each playing its specialized role in the maintenance of good health and efficient function, that to speak of disease of an individual organ is to suggest an autonomy that is undeserved. If one organ malfunctions, it is likely that there will be repercussions in most other systems.

Robert W. Boxer, M.D.

U *pdate on candida testing and treatment (2001):*

I routinely use the candida immune complexes from AAL Lab and we find that there are very few false positives. Generally when the values are elevated, the patients do respond to anti-yeast treatment. There are some false negatives, and I suspect it is anywhere between 20 all the way up to 40% at times. So I will still use my clinical judgment; i.e. if I suspect the patient has a yeast problem, I will treat him, because the treatment is so safe, particularly if we stay with nystatin, diet, probiotics and other supplements.

If the test is negative, I may do a stool for comprehensive parasitology and bacteriology through Great Smokies and if this is 3 or 4+, I think that is also good evidence that the patient probably has yeast imbalance.

We have been using nystatin tablets in some patients who don't or won't take the powder four times a day. It seems to be awfully important to take some form of nystatin four times a day. For those people who are so much on the run that they can't, using the tablets especially at lunchtime, is helpful. It is a little bit of a compromise but I think we are avoiding winning the battle and losing the war by doing this.

I have a few patients who take the tablets only and they

have improved also. Obviously the tablets have excipients, such as fillers, binders and dyes and they don't work in the mouth, throat or the esophagus, but nevertheless they probably are about 80% as effective (just as a rough guess), and most of the patients are using the powder mainly or exclusively.

We do have some patients on amphotericin B, 100 mg four times a day and it is a little too early to evaluate progress, but so far I'm not that impressed. I may have had one patient who had a true allergic reaction to the amphotericin B, even at that dose. It is not supposed to be absorbed at that dose.

I obtain baseline lab studies on patients because I think anybody on chronic medication should probably have baseline labs. If there are any abnormalities in liver or kidney function or blood count, then I will repeat them after a month. Of course, when I put patients on Diflucan or Sporanox, I do lab studies very frequently and track them so that I can pick up trends toward abnormalities even before the values become actually abnormal.

Out of about 300 patients we have treated with azole antifungals, we have picked up five patients who clearly were having a problem because of the antifungal and we stopped it. The abnormal lab results were reversed in almost the same order in which they appeared with the same time sequence, suggesting a cause and effect relationship.

I hope this update helps and that you're having a great summer.

With kind personal regards,

Sincerely,

Bob

James H. Brodsky, M.D.

I n the *Foreword* to the third edition of **The Yeast Connection** (1986), Dr. Brodsky made these remarks.

It is time for all physicians and medical scientists to increase their understanding of the relationship between yeast and human illness. Many patients with yeast-related health disorders are being treated ineffectively just because their problem has gone unrecognized.

If one reviews the literature carefully, the supporting research is well documented. Antibiotics have been shown to inhibit both antibody synthesis and phagocytic activity, and thus may reduce the host resistance to invasion by *Candida albicans*. Once established, candida components further depress immune function. Mannan, a carbohydrate component of candida, inhibits human lymphocyte proliferation.

Taking sera from women with recurrent vaginal candidiasis, Witkin and associates, were able to demonstrate a reduced or absent lymphocyte response to candida antigens. In another paper, Witkin thoroughly reviews the defective immune response in patients with recurrent candida infections.

The literature, therefore, clearly supports the the-

ory that antibiotics can lead to candida overgrowth which suppresses immune function thereby predisposing one to recurrent infections. (emphasis added) There is much evidence to suggest that *C. albicans* is one of the most allergenic microbes. Both immediate and delayed hypersensitivity reactions to candida are very common in the adult population.

The relationship between yeast and urticaria has been established in a well-designed double blind trial. The investigators estimate that in about 26% of patients with chronic urticaria, *C. albicans* sensitivity is an important factor. Significant clinical improvement was seen with anti-candida therapy and a low-yeast diet.

An increase in the population of *C. albicans* following antibiotic therapy or change in diet may also cause a chronic "irritable bowel" syndrome. This is ascribed to hypersensitivity to the organism or its metabolic products rather than actual infection. *C. albicans* can cause allergic reactions in the large bowel and other mucous membranes. The work of Holti was so compelling that it was referenced in two of the most respected texts dealing with candida.

The importance of the role of the intestinal tract in treating patients with recurrent vulvovaginal candidiasis has been nearly ignored. Vaginal candidiasis does not occur without the concomitant presence of *C. albicans* within the large bowel and a cure is unlikely as long as the vagina remains the only treatment target.

Enteric candida undoubtedly play a greater role in human illness than has been previously suspected. A history of food and chemical intolerances is frequently seen in patients with a history of recurrent candida infections. There is increasing evidence that gut yeast may have a role in some cases of psoriasis. Changes in mood and behavior related to yeast have been observed for over 30 years and are reviewed by Iwata. Health professionals must take note of what is known about the yeast-human interactions. We must help our patients overcome this illness, which is probably, for most, iatrogenic* in origin.

Here are excerpts from his Foreword to **The Yeast Connection and the Woman** *(1995/1997/1998).*

Since *The Yeast Connection* was first published in 1983, many new ideas have appeared relative to the role of yeast in human illness. During the past decade, the number of patients who have been diagnosed and successfully treated have been legion. Patient testimonies, many of which are cited in this text, are compelling. They have encouraged those of us who treat this and related disorders to continue our efforts . . . The book cites countless references for those who wish to read further about how the yeast theory evolved, what evidence supports it, and what treatments appear to be effective.

During the past decade, we have learned a great deal about chronic fatigue and the importance of listening to and not dismissing patients who complain of it. Many individuals with chronic fatigue immune dysfunction syndrome

---

*Iatrogenic means induced inadvertently by the medical treatment or procedures of a physician.

(CFIDS) have responded well to treatment for yeast, suggesting there may be a relationship between yeast and this illness. Cognitive impairment, sometimes described as spaciness, poor memory, or loss of concentration, is an all too common complaint. After other causes of this have been systematically excluded, a trial of yeast-reduction therapy is suggested and is often remarkably effective.

Other common problems such as allergy, irritable bowel syndrome, PMS, depression and fibromyalgia may also have a relationship to yeast. It has been suggested that certain autoimmune disorders and less common problems such as interstitial cystitis and vulvodynia may be related to yeast since they frequently respond to yeast-reduction therapy. If there is a relationship between these common and not so common disorders and yeast, then this must be better defined and acknowledged. The health of many depends on it.

✦✦✦ ✉ ✦✦✦

Dr. Brodsky is a Diplomate of the American Board of Internal Medicine and a clinical instructor at Georgetown Medical Center. He lives in the Washington, DC area. I've seen him numerous times in the last 18 years and have sought his advice and counsel about my patients. He has also provided information for my books and lectures.

Dr. Crook

John Curlin, M.D.

 n pages 173–174 of my 1986 book, **The Yeast Connection,** I included these comments of Jackson, Tennessee, gynecologist, Dr. Curlin.

Since entering practice, I've seen thousands of patients with symptoms related to hormone dysfunction. Their complaints have included pelvic pain, menstrual irregularities, PMS (premenstrual syndrome), infertility, nausea and vomiting of pregnancy, endometriosis, vaginitis, painful intercourse and absence of normal sexual interest and responsiveness.

Three years ago I learned of the observations of Joseph Miller and Richard Mabray who noted that women who experienced painful menstruation, premenstrual syndrome and other symptoms of hormone dysfunction often responded to tiny doses of progesterone. I began to use this method of therapy in patients in my own practice and found that many of them improved, often dramatically.

Then two years ago I learned about yeast-related illness and began to use diet, nystatin and candida extracts in treating these patients. Although this program doesn't relieve all of the symptoms caused by hormone dysfunction, the response in most of my patients has been gratifying. In addition to the "typical" gynecological problems that have responded, many patients with other health problems, including arthritis, colitis and other auto-immune disorders, have also improved.

In discussing health problems of children, on page 196 of the same book, I again cited the comments of Dr. Curlin who said,

My 13-year-old daughter is a well-coordinated gymnast. However, since infancy, she had showed periods of depression and fatigue. And during the past year or so, she has noticed periodic changes in her ability to concentrate and coordinate her movements.

During the past year, we've learned that **she does extremely well if she maintains her diet and nystatin therapy.** If she does not, her moodiness and marked fatigue will return. And, interestingly, she'll show a lack of physical coordination in her gymnastics.

Our youngest son, now 14 months of age, was fed only breast milk during his first six months of life and continued on breast milk plus other foods until the age of one year. Nevertheless, he was constantly irritable and suffered from a chronic rhinitis.

Almost within 24 hours after I began giving him small doses of nystatin powder, his rhinitis cleared and he showed a noticeable change in personality. His irritability subsided and he became much more pleasant.

This is so impressive that family members can recognize when his daily doses of nystatin have been forgotten by the sudden changes in his behavior. Then when he receives his nystatin, he settles down.

In the spring of 1993, I was invited to give a presentation to a group of gynecologists at the University of Tennessee. In gathering information, I again asked Dr. Curlin for his observations and comments. Here's an excerpt from a letter he sent me.

Since you stimulated my interest over 15 years ago, I've treated literally hundreds of patients with oral nystatin, sugar-free diet and emphasis on good health measures such as exercise . . .

If a patient is willing to abide by the diet and take the nystatin, recurrent vaginal candidiasis can be successfully treated almost 100% of the time. And many patients with chronic fatigue and multiple other immune dysfunction symptoms can also be greatly helped.

In talking to my patients I tell them of the controversy regarding the causes of the symptoms and the treatment. Yet, I've had no adverse effect from the therapy and many patients who found no relief in the orthodox medical community have been greatly helped by this simple therapy.

✦✦✦ ✉ ✦✦✦

Since that time, Dr. Curlin has retired from his general practice of gynecology and until recently served as a member of the Advisory Board of the International Health Foundation.

Dr. Crook

Carol Jessop, M.D.*

O n April 15, 1989 a conference on CFS sponsored by the University of California Medical Center and other professional organizations was held in San Francisco. In her presentation at this conference, Dr. Jessop described her observations on 1,100 patients with CFS. Here's a reference to Dr. Jessop's presentation published in **American Medical News,** May 26, 1989.

Internist Carol Jessop, a private practitioner in El Cerrito, California, who is following 1100 patients with CFS, believes the illness would be more aptly called "chronic devastation syndrome!" In many instances, said Dr. Jessop, CFS patients became so ill that they had to crawl to the bathroom.

According to Dr. Jessop, 80% of her patients had recurrent ear, nose and throat infections as children; had acne as adolescents; had recurrent hives, anxiety attacks, headaches and bowel problems; and had to stop drinking alcohol because it didn't agree with them. Ninety percent had cholesterol levels higher than 225.

---

*Diplomate, American Board of Internal Medicine Assistant Clinical Professor of Medicine, University of California, San Francisco, American College of Physicians, American Society of Internal Medicine.

Beginning last year, Dr. Jessop treated 900 of her CFS patients with ketoconazole, a drug used to treat candidiasis, and placed them on a sugar-free diet. Since then, 529 have returned to their previous health and another 232 have shown improvement, she said.

Dr. Jessop said that her patients have taught her about CFS. *"I didn't learn it in medical school,"* she added.

She urged more physicians to listen to complaints from fatigued patients. *"It's important that the patients feel they're in control,"* she said.

If patients are also seeking help from alternative health practitioners, such as body workers or acupuncturists, Dr. Jessop says she doesn't discourage them.

Often she says such patients "feel abandoned" by the traditional medical community. *"Keep up a dialogue"* with your patients, Dr. Jessop urged.

I attended this conference, along with 500 professionals and nonprofessionals. Other speakers at the conference included Paul Cheney, M.D., Ph.D., James F. Jones, M.D., Anthony Komaroff, M.D. and J. A. Levy, M.D.

I met Dr. Jessop at the conference and I was excited to hear her presentation. The following day I had dinner with Dr. Jessop and several other San Francisco physicians. Dr. Jessop and I continued our friendship and she wrote the following Foreword of my 1992 book **Chronic Fatigue Syndrome and the Yeast Connection.***

---

*This book was replaced in 2001 by my book, *Tired—So Tired!* and the "yeast connection."

This book does not claim that the common yeast, *Candida albicans,* is the cause of CFS. However, it does explain the role of multiple entities: yeast overgrowth, intestinal parasites, unchecked viral infections, food allergies and chemical sensitivities—and how these can result in the immune dysregulation we refer to as CFS.

Chronic Fatigue Syndrome (CFS) is a devastating illness which has affected young and middle-aged people in increasing proportions over the past few decades. Epidemic and endemic reports of this illness and the number of affected patients seem to be rising steadily. Most clinicians working with CFS believe it is unlikely that one cause, or for example one virus, is responsible for this syndrome.

Having worked with CFS patients for almost 10 years, I believe this illness may simply represent the 10 to 15% of our species who have not yet adapted to the rapid and startling changes in the environment, and the subsequent changes in our internal intestinal environment.

Since 1950 we've seen the development and overuse of antibiotics; the use of hormones and birth control pills; the development of immunosuppressive drugs; the introduction of various chemicals and toxins into our environment; and significant changes which have occurred within our diets, leaving us foods tainted with pesticides, depleted in nutritional value and loaded with sugars and dyes.

Can we really continue to believe these incredible changes have not affected the well-being of some and eventually perhaps all of us?

In this book, Dr. Crook reviews information presented at medical conferences and published in medical journals which discuss the correlation of intestinal yeast overgrowth and resultant toxic and immunological effects. He makes suggestions to patients which help them clarify whether food allergies, candida or mineral deficiencies are contributing to their illness.

Many of the suggestions in this book will prove most helpful to my patients. The use of antifungal medication is becoming more common among clinicians treating CFS patients and nutritional supplements are gaining widespread support. Clinicians who are overwhelmed by patients with multiple systemic complaints may find that having their patients read this book will guide them toward a more stable course in their illness.

Ten years ago I was very frustrated working with CFS patients because of deeply ingrained skepticism about theories such as the "yeast connection." However, following further research and a trial of some of these therapeutic interventions with my patients, my work has become both intellectually rewarding and fun.

Hopefully this book will be the springboard to help many clinicians and patients understand this devastating illness.

•• •• •• ✉ •• •• ••

Dr. Jessop moved on from her practice of internal medicine and I haven't corresponded with her in the last few years. According to mutual friends, she's now serving on the staff of a California hospital.

Dr. Crook

Donald Lewis, M.D.

I n my 1995 book, **The Yeast Connection and the Woman,** I included these comments of Jackson, Tennessee, gynecologist, Dr. Lewis.

After the initial skepticism, I decided to try the diet/nystatin approach . . . as much out of desperation as for other reasons . . . I was initially amazed and subsequently quite gratified to know that I did have an approach that promised success to a fairly large subset of my patients.

If I might add, that it has also been interesting to talk with the patients one or two months into the program. When I inquire about their vaginitis symptoms, they frequently say, *"Oh yes, that's better. But the greatest thing is my sinuses have opened up for the first time in several years."*

So there are obviously other side benefits that can be gained from this approach that are far afield from the initial reason for treatment.

✦✦✦ ⊠ ✦✦✦

Don, a board certified obstetrician and gynecologist, moved to Jackson in the 1960s and joined the Woman's Clinic. He became a friend of mine and after helping many, many people for 30 years, he retired in July 2001.

Dr. Crook

Heiko Santelmann, M.D.

Sven, a funny and positive man, met in my office for the first time when he was 42 years old. But he looked older. He had gray hair and trouble with his knees. He walked like they were stiff and swollen. When I shook his hand, I noted that his fingers were bent and understood that he was suffering from severe rheumatism. He had been working in an office until he could not hold a pen anymore, and that was at an age of 40.

Sven told me he had been tired for many years but that he never was seriously ill or hospitalized until he was 35. He got several infections the last years, in the throat, the sinuses, the lungs and urine bladder. A few weeks after one infection was successfully treated by antibiotics, another infection popped up. Soon he was suffering from fungal infections as well. He was itching in his ears and around his anus and his tongue was coated with a white layer of candida.

When Sven was complaining about abdominal discomfort after all these antibiotics, he got his stomach checked. The tests showed that there were HP-bacteria present, a type which could cause stomach ulcers, and he was put on a regimen with three very strong antibiotics at the same time. A few months later his lymph nodes were swollen and painful "without a reason." He could not see and hear as good as before, his gums were infected and he was bothered with lots of mucus in his throat.

Two months after that he developed rheumatoid arthritis. He got severe pain and swellings in almost all of his joints, but his knees were worse, they became big as footballs, Sven explained. The specialists had no doubt about the diagnosis and the blood test results were also typical. They tried lots of different medicines, NSAIDs like Voltaren, Brufen, Brexidol, cortisone, Salazopyrin and even cytostatics, but the side effects were serious and he had to stop them.

Two years later he went to his doctor because of an eczema that looked like psoriasis. But the doctor suspected an infection and prescribed three weeks with antibiotics. Under this treatment his rheumatism and other problems increased, he got fungus infections between his toes and on some fingernails and he started wondering if his problems were yeast-related. He found out that his joints were less swollen and painful when he dropped eating sugar and honey and that he reacted with diarrhea to lactose. He also tried a natural antibiotic, grapeseed extract, but already after just a few days with 5 drops, he got a reaction of panic anxiety and stopped. He started with tea tree oil instead, 5 to 10 drops twice a day, which he tolerated good. He realized a slight improvement under that treatment.

When Sven came to my office, I took an allergy skin test for *Candida albicans* on his arm, which was positive. But since a 2-weeks test-diet without yeasts, molds, milk and sugar only improved his symptoms marginally, I had to look for other factors as well. When I found out that he had an allergic reaction to wristwatches with nickel, I asked him if he ever had observed a negative reaction after visiting his dentist. And so he had. Already since he was 12 years old, he got sick with an infection almost every time after he had visited the dentist. The correlation was obvious.

Now Sven wanted to get his mercury-containing tooth fillings removed and contacted a dentist who had special equipment to secure a removing of the amalgam without letting him inhale the dust and gas. He also took lots of vitamins and minerals. But in spite of that, Sven's joints got worse for 2–3 days each time he had one filling removed.

Finally, after all his fillings were removed, I prescribed a chelating medicine, DMSA, to get the mercury out of his body as well. But even a very low dose made him depressed for several days. When I gave him some drops of a homeopathic formula instead, his joints reacted and he got a headache.

After all these years with pain and lots of other problems, my patient became impatient. He had removed his mercury fillings, he knew he had fungus infections and an allergy against *Candida albicans* and his yeast-related problems had increased during this time. He wanted to get rid of the candida now, not after the DMSA cure. So I gave him a prescription for one capsule of 150 mg Diflucan (fluconazole), a fast acting, systemic antifungal medication, as a test. This one pill decreased the inflammation in several of his joints for one week. He was thrilled!—And so was I.

He got a new prescription and took 150 mg every second

day for two weeks. This made his headache blow away, the pain in the joints decreased again and he felt relaxed 2 hours after each capsule. When he walked into my office after these 2 weeks, he walked straight, normal and quick, and when he shook my hand, the fingers were stretched out. At a first glance there were no signs of rheumatism any more.— I had never seen such a big improvement of a rheumatic arthritis in such a short time without high doses of cortisone.

Sven got an antimycotic oil complex, ("Oregano Complex" from Biocare, UK), two capsules every day, and when he had money enough, also Diflucan. But when he stopped the Diflucan for more than 2 weeks, his joints began to hurt and swell again. Also when he dropped his diet, he got a relapse. Over some weeks he tried 300mg Diflucan 2 times a week, got very much better, but again worse 2 weeks later.

Now he understood that it was necessary to clean the body for mercury first. Sven started again with the DMSA treatment, slowly, 100mg every second to fourth week. When he could not register any side effects of the cleansing any more, he increased the dose to 200mg, and so on. Sometimes his stools got a strong gray color, sometimes his joints reacted, sometimes he got depressed and sometimes he got his eczema back. But his health was improving. The days between the DMSA he was taking Chlorella algae or L-Cystein together with his antioxidants and probiotics.

The last time I met Sven, he walked almost normally, his joints were only a little bit swollen, even if he had not taken Diflucan for several months. He told me that it sometimes feels like clouds are vanishing from his forehead and that he can think more clearly after taking the DMSA, but that he still had not taken the maximum dose I prescribed. "I have not had one infection after I started your treatment" he said.

His family and friends were very surprised about his improvement. He showed me his hair, which was all gray and straight before. Now it was getting more and more black again, and curly. He looked more than ten years younger now and has trouble explaining to others that this is a result of the treatment of a doctor and not of a hairdresser.

Sven has not finished his detoxification treatment yet. But I am very excited to see how much better he will get after most of the mercury is removed from his body. He is supposed to increase the DMSA dose to 100mg 3 times a day for 3 days every 3rd week and continue for several months, until he doesn't register any negative or positive reactions any more. Thereafter he has to take some DMPS, another chelating medicine, before it is time for a new cure with a high dose of Diflucan.

In my opinion, it probably was the amalgam from his fillings, which harmed his immune system and caused the recurrent infections in the first place. Than he developed allergy to the increasing amount of yeasts due to the massive doses of antibiotics. And this allergy could have started his arthritis. The test proved that he was suffering from Candida-Related Complex, but in order to get well and stay well without having to continue with antimycotics and diet for years, it was vital to get the mercury removed from his fillings and body.—But another very important reason for his improvement is his positive attitude to life, his strong belief and will to get well again, despite the bad prognoses from the specialists.

Dr. Heiko Santelmann MD
Oslo, 20.08.2001

✻✻✻ ✉ ✻✻✻

*Dr. Santelmann is a remarkable person. I say this for many reasons. Here are some of them. He is smart and persistent. He began working to get a scientific study published on nystatin in the 1980s. It was published in a peer-reviewed British journal in 2001. He translated the paperback edition of **The Yeast Connection** into Norwegian.*

Heiko has been my friend for many years. I sat on the porch of an Oslo hotel with him for four hours some nine years ago while my wife and I were on a Baltic cruise. He also has served as a member of the Advisory Board of the International Health Foundation for many years.

Dr. Crook

Paul Schwartz, M.D.

ere's a copy of a letter which was sent to me over eight years ago by a physician in my community.

September 29, 1993

Dear Dr. Crook:

Just a note to bring you up to date with my current practice.

Since having the opportunity to work with you in the early spring of 1981, I have seen numerous patients who have been helped by some of the dietary manipulations and yeast treatment that you have preached for so many years.

One young patient who comes to mind is a boy in the 3rd grade that I saw about 7–8 years ago who was to the point of being sent home from school. His mother was a 5th grade teacher in the same school and he was a highly intelligent young man who simply could not sit still. After approximately three weeks of following the pattern in your original book on tracking down hidden food allergies, the young man and his mother presented back to my office. When I asked how things were, his mother deferred to the young man sitting on the exam table and said, "tell him."

At this point the young man grinned ear to ear and said, "*I have not had near as many whippings.*" The mother indicated that he had very significant reactions when challenged with corn syrup and with ketchup. This young man, with very minimal dietary manipulations and restrictions, went on to have a very successful school year and his behavioral problems resolved considerably. Obviously both mother, child and school teachers were thrilled with such a simple solution.

I continue to see patients from time to time who meet a significant number of the suggested criteria for chronic candidiasis. Some of these are members of my own family who have suffered depression and considerable fatigue along with gastrointestinal symptoms of flatulence and pain. Many of these patients have seen very significant reaction when changing their diet and utilizing some of the anti-candidal therapy.

I hope at sometime, some academician will be able to take the information that you have worked to glean over a lifetime of frontline research and put it in a form that will be intellectually acceptable to the rest of the medical community. In the meantime, I am proud to have worked with you and continue to utilize some of these modalities of treatment that provide some relief to patients that have been basically ignored by much of the medical profession.

Paul E. Schwartz, M.D.
Jackson Clinic
Department of Family Medicine

✸✸✸ ✉ ✸✸✸

Dr. Schwartz spent several weeks with me and my colleagues at the Children's Clinic when he was a resident physician in the

University of Tennessee Department of Family Medicine. He's a skilled and experienced physician and a dedicated and compassionate man who has helped many, many patients. I regret to say that he's the only one of the over 300 physicians in practice in my community who has expressed a significant interest in yeast-related problems.

Dr. Crook

Ray C. Wunderlich, Jr., M.D.

I n my 1986 book, **The Yeast Connection,** in a two-page statement entitled, "A Special Message for the Physician," I included the comments of this Florida physician who said,

Desirable at all times, is a balanced approach that holds a healthy respect of *Candida albicans* . . . At the same time, one does not wish to overlook the many other health departures that invite the candida syndrome. Those who suspect that they have symptoms due to candida overgrowth must not plunge headlong into a quest for a 'magic bullet.' Best and most long lasting health will be fostered by a careful inquiry into yeast, but also, into psychological, nutritional, allergic, degenerative and toxic factors.

During the past 14 years, Wunderlich and I have discussed our interests and observations in person, by mail and on the phone. I've been pleased because for several decades he's written about food allergies and the adverse effects of consuming sugar. He's also shared with me his own observations in managing his patients.

*In 1997, he published a superb 48-page booklet, **The Candida-Yeast Syndrome**—The spreading epidemic of yeast-connected diseases: how to recognize and deal with them. Here are excerpts from his introduction.*

The yeast connection now occupies center stage in the practices of nutritionally oriented doctors, nutritionists and many other therapists who see clearly the broad range of factors that account for so much of the misery that their clients experience. For better or worse, health food store personnel have become resident experts on the condition because of the flock of individuals who patronize their stores seeking relief when their doctors fail to provide help or brand them as hysterical, neurotic or misguided.

Thus . . . we have a vastly informed public at the same time the bulk of the standard medical profession fails to recognize the yeast syndrome as a bona fide condition . . . It is a complex of conditions, a disease process that may be a primary or secondary disorder. The yeast overgrowth complex, silent or evident, usually manifests itself in the gastrointestinal tract. It is one of those conditions . . . that often quietly produces over the years a load of unwanted chemicals, toxins, macromolecules or partially digested foods that, in turn, adversely impact the liver and other target organs . . . All this usually occurs gradually over months, years, even decades of life . . .

As one studies the yeast connection, one is struck by the rampant side effects of the chemical, dietary and antibiotic assaults made upon us since the industrial revolution, the introduction of processed foods and the medical profession's love affair with antibiotics. Lest I come across as a radical nihilist in human affairs, let me assert that the march of progress of civilization has at the same time provided us with amazing benefits. Yet I recognize too the enormous price that each of us has paid and is paying for the advances of civilization. Part of that price is the yeast complex.

Martin H. Zwerling, M.D.*

There are not such things as incurables, there are only things for which man has not found a cure.   —Baruch

C onsider the following "incurable" patient, who is being treated by several specialists. Her gynecologist is treating her recurrent vaginitis and irregular menstrual periods, while an otolaryngologist is trying to control her external otitis and chronic rhinitis. At the same time, her internist is unsuccessfully attempting to manage symptoms of bloating, indigestion and abdominal pain, and a dermatologist is struggling with bizarre skin rashes, hives and psoriasis. Lastly, her psychiatrist has been unable to convince the patient that her "nerves" are the cause of her extreme irritability, inability to concentrate and depression.

We have all been guilty of labeling such patients as "psychosomatic" and since there is "nothing physically wrong," conclude we can not cure them.

Incurable? Not if you THINK YEAST. This patient and thousands like her are suffering from chronic candidiasis.

---

*This discussion comes from a 1984 article in the *Journal of the South Carolina Medical Association* by Dr. Zwerling and two of his colleagues, Kenneth N. Owens, M.D. and Nancy H. Ruth, R.N., B.S.

Over the last forty years, new advances in medicine have permitted the candida to proliferate in certain patients. These recent medical developments are:

1. Antibiotics by prescription and also in our food supply can upset the normal gastrointestinal flora and favor the growth of yeast within us.
2. Steroids and immune-suppressant drugs stimulate the growth of Candida albicans.
3. Oral contraceptives as well as frequent pregnancies can cause an imbalance of hormones which favor overgrowth of Candida.

To these medical advances should be added the recent increased consumption of yeasty foods such as bread, wine, cheeses and mushrooms, which add to the imbalance in favor of yeasts.

Symptoms

Most of the symptoms of chronic candidiasis affect three main parts of the body.

Intestinal and Genital Urinary Systems

Menstrual complaints, vaginitis, abdominal discomfort, distension, constipation, rectal itching, cystitis and urethritis.

Nervous System

Severe depression, extreme irritability, inability to concentrate, headaches and memory lapses.

Allergy and Immune Systems

Asthma, hay fever, external otitis, urticaria, and severe sensitivities to tobacco, smoke, perfumes, diesel fumes and other chemical odors.

Diagnosis

Candida albicans is present in every individual, and anti-IgE for candida is present in 100 percent of humans. Most patients can have a culture of candida grown from their mouth or intestinal tract, and it only requires forty-eight hours on tetracycline to easily culture candida from all individuals. Therefore, with cultures, skin testing, RAST testing and serology unable to differentiate between a well person and one in whom candida is causing disease, diagnosis is often difficult. However, if we train ourselves to THINK YEAST, then the diagnosis should be suspected by an appropriate history and confirmed by a therapeutic trial.

Report of Cases

From January, 1979 to January, 1984, a group of 79 patients with chronic candidiasis were treated. There were 53 women and 26 men, and all the patients were from the private practices of the authors. The most common complaints were for chronic vaginitis, external otitis and allergic dermatitis. Many of the patients had combinations of symptoms and it was rare to find a female patient with chronic vaginitis who did not also have bloating, mental depression or rash.

The first 35 patients were treated by desensitization alone. Later, as more knowledge was gained, the use of a yeast-restricted diet, anti-fungal medication and restriction of etiological causes (such as antibiotics, steroids and birth control pills) were added to the therapy. The best results were obtained by combining all four treatments.

Results

Of the 79 patients treated, 70 had good to excellent results. Four patients dropped out of the study and were lost to follow-up. Five patients had no improvement in their symptoms and these therapeutic failures were considered cases of non-candidiasis and further diagnostic studies were ordered.

Special Comment

In the course of this study, it occurred to one of the authors (M.H.Z.) that the role *Candida albicans* played in making "poor old Charlie Swaart" drunk, could also explain a common and up to now, untreatable ENT complaint, bad breath. just as the "still" in Charlie Swaart's stomach was converting carbohydrates directly into alcohol, it was thought that possibly the candida could also ferment other foods in the stomach and was converting carbohydrates directly into alcohol, it was thought that possibly the candida could also ferment other foods in the stomach and cause halitosis (bad breath).

In a busy ENT practice it is not difficult to find patients

with intractable bad breath, most of whom have had their tonsils and teeth removed, along with assorted abdominal organs, in unsuccessful attempts for relief. Fifteen patients with halitosis were placed on the therapeutic trial (avoidance of sugar and foods rich in yeast and mold, elimination of antibiotics, steroids and birth-control pills, killing of yeast cells with nystatin and/or ketoconazole).

Within 24 to 48 hours, all fifteen patients reported marked improvements in their breath odor and this was confirmed by their families and the examining physician. This is the first report of the use of anti-yeast treatment in halitosis.

Conclusion

Dr. William G. Crook, in his excellent book, *The Yeast Connection*, concludes by stating: *"Since I first learned of the relationship of Candida albicans to human illness, my life and my practice have changed dramatically. I can hardly wait to get to my office each day because I know I'll be seeing people I can help. Many of them complain of so many symptoms they've been labeled 'hypochondriacs.'"*

Others with supposedly incurable diseases have been told, *"You'll have to learn to live with this condition."* Yet, in the last four years, I've been able to help hundreds of long-suffering adult patients. Moreover, my experiences are being duplicated by many other physicians.

This paper confirms that some of the sickest patients seen in private practice have a problem with *Candida albi-*

cans, and will respond to treatment. Fifteen patients with intractable halitosis were successfully controlled by anti-candida treatment.

••• ⊠ •••

*I read the article by Martin Zwerling and colleagues about a year after it was published. I was excited—even thrilled—to read it. I included a reference to this article in **The Yeast Connection and the Woman** (1995), **The Yeast Connection Handbook** (1997) and **Tired—So Tired! and the "yeast connection"** (2001). In each of these books I included a copy of the first page of Dr. Zwerling's 1984 article. It still ranks at the top of the list of articles about Candida albicans that are easy to read and understand.*

*Martin continues to be in practice and we exchanged many letters. Recently he sent me a copy of the July 2001 issue of the **Journal of the South Carolina Medical Association** and I was pleased to see that he was the guest editor.*

Dr. Crook

☑

SHORT QUESTIONNAIRE

Are Your Health Problems Yeast Connected?

Questionnaire

I f your answer is "yes" to any question circle the number in the right-hand column. When you've completed the questionnaire, add up the points you've circled. Your score will help you determine the possibility (or probability) that your health problems are yeast connected.

	YES	NO	SCORE
1. Have you taken repeated or prolonged courses of antibacterial drugs?	☐	☐	4
2. Have you been bothered by recurrent vaginal, prostate or urinary infections?	☐	☐	3
3. Do you feel "sick all over," yet the cause hasn't been found?	☐	☐	2
4. Are you bothered by hormone disturbances, including PMS, menstrual irregularities, sexual dysfunction, sugar craving, low body temperature or fatigue?	☐	☐	2
5. Are you unusually sensitive to tobacco smoke, perfumes, colognes and other chemical odors?	☐	☐	2

	YES	NO	SCORE
6. Are you bothered by memory or concentration problems? Do you sometimes feel "spaced out?"	☐	☐	2
7. Have you taken prolonged courses of prednisone or other steroids; or have you taken "the pill" for more than 3 years?	☐	☐	2
8. Do some foods disagree with you or trigger your symptoms?	☐	☐	1
9. Do you suffer with constipation, diarrhea, bloating or abdominal pain?	☐	☐	1
10. Does your skin itch, tingle or burn; or is it unusually dry; or are you bothered by rashes?	☐	☐	1

Scoring for women: If your score is 9 or more, your health problems are probably yeast connected. If your score is 12 or more, your health problems are almost certainly yeast connected.

Scoring for men: If your score is 7 or more, your health problems are probably yeast connected. If your score is 10 or more, your health problems are almost certainly yeast connected.

Other Sources of Information and Help

D iflucan can be obtained on prescription from any pharmacy. At this time, prescriptions of sugar-free oral nystatin powder can only be obtained from a few pharmacies, including:.

The Apothecary, Bethesda, MD 20814, 800-869-9159, Fax: 301-493-4671.

Bio Tech Pharmacal, Fayetteville, AR, 72702, 800-345-1199, Fax: 501-443-5643

College Pharmacy, Colorado Springs, Co, 80903, 800-888-9356, Fax: 800-556-5893.

Freeda Pharmacy, New York, NY, 10017, 800-777-3737, Fax: 212-685-7297.

Hopewell Pharmacy and Compounding, Hopewell, NJ 08525, 800-792-6670, Fax: 800-417-3864.

Medical Towers Pharmacy, Birmingham, AL 35205, 800-378-7877 or 205-933-7381.

N.E.E.D.S., Syracuse, NY 13209, 800-634-1380, Fax: 315-488-6336.

Wellness Health and Pharmaceuticals, Birmingham, AL 35209, 800-227-2627, Fax: 800-369-0302.

Willner Chemist, New York, NY 10017, 800-633-1106, Fax: 212-682-6192.

Women's International Pharmacy, 5708 Monona Dr., Madison, WI 53716-3152, 800-279-5708, Fax: 800-279-8011.

Nonprescription agents and nutritional supplements used by many people whose stories are in this book can be obtained from the pharmacies listed above, your health food store and from other sources, including:

Douglas Laboratories, 800-245-4440 or 888-368-4522; www.douglaslabs.com; e-mail: nutrition@douglaslabs.com

Swanson Health Products, 800-437-4148, www.swanson vitamins.com

East Park Research, P.O. Box 530099, Henderson, NV 89053.

Internet Sources:

www.candida-yeast.com
www.greatplainslaboratory.com
www.imbris/7Emastent7E
www.candidapage.com
www.savorypalate.com
www.nlci.com/nutrition
www.cssa-inc.org
www.hhi.org
www.drmagaziner.com
www.drcranton.com
www.wellnesshealth.com

www.cfs-recovery.org
www.parentsofallergicchildren.org
www.needs.com
www.alternativementalhealth.com
www.sbakermd.com
www.mdheal.org
www.geocities.com/HotSprings/2125
www.CassMD.com
www.vitalitydoctor.com
www.swansonvitamins.com
www.eastparkresearch
www.kolorex

About the Author

W illiam G. Crook, M.D., received his medical education and training at the University of Virginia, the Pennsylvania Hospital, Vanderbilt and Johns Hopkins. He is an Emeritus Fellow of the American Academy of Pediatrics, the American College of Allergy, Asthma and Immunology and the American Academy of Environmental Medicine. He is a member of the American Medical Association, the American Academy of Allergy and Immunology, Alpha Omega Alpha and other medical organizations.

Dr. Crook is the author of 14 previous books and numerous reports in the medical and lay literature. For fifteen years he wrote a nationally syndicated health column, "Child Care" (*General Features* and the *Los Angeles Times* Syndicates).

Various of his publications have been translated into French, German, Japanese and Norwegian.

Yeast Connection Success Stories is the seventh in his series of books which deal with the relationship of *Candida albicans* to many puzzling health disorders. The titles include *The Yeast Connection, Chronic Fatigue Syndrome and the Yeast Connection, The Yeast Connection Handbook,* and *Tired—So Tired! and the yeast connection.*

Dr. Crook has been a popular guest on local, regional,

national and international television and radio programs, including the BBC, Good Morning Australia, Oprah Winfrey, Regis Philbin, Sally Jessy Raphael, The 700 Club, and TV Ontario.

He has addressed professional and lay groups in 39 states, all Canadian provinces, Australia, England, Italy, Malaysia, Mexico, The Netherlands, New Zealand and Venezuela. And he has served as a visiting professor at Ohio State University, and the Universities of California (San Francisco) and Saskatchewan.

Dr. Crook lives in Jackson, Tennessee, with his wife, Betsy. They have three daughters and four grandchildren. His interests include helping people, golf, bridge, oil painting and travel.

Suggestions for Further Reading

ommenting on *The Yeast Connection Handbook,* James H. Brodsky, M.D., Diplomate, American Board of Internal Medicine, said,

> "An extraordinary handbook and resource guide for individuals with yeast-related illness. With remarkable simplicity, Dr. Crook gives us an approach to many health problems overlooked by conventional medicine. *It should be read by every person who is not well and unable to find help.*"

To learn more about foods you can eat and how to prepare them, get a copy of *The Yeast Connection Cookbook* which includes over 200 recipes. Here's an excerpt from the introduction of co-author, Marjorie Hurt Jones, R.N.:

> "I've emphasized tasty vegetables of all sorts which will make your diet more enjoyable and less apt to cause allergies . . . I can't deny that cooking takes time, *I can only suggest that, if you really want to enjoy better health, planning and preparing nutritious meals is the place to start.*"

Commenting on *Tired—So Tired!* and the *"yeast connection,"* Martie Whittiken, Certified Clinical Nutritionist, Vital Nutrition, Dallas, Texas, said,

"This book is written for average Americans with an energy crisis. Instead of popping pills folks should read *Tired - So Tired!* and learn that the fatigue is a blessing in disguise. It is warning them they're on a slippery slope toward more serious health problems. As always, Dr. Crook not only gives us a wake up call, but practical help and many useful resources. This book will be assigned as homework for many of my clients."

New Information For
The Twenty-First Century!

THE
YEAST
CONNECTION
HANDBOOK

How Yeasts Can Make You Feel
"Sick All Over"
and the Steps *You* Need
to Take to Regain *Your* Health

William G. Crook, M.D.

THE
YEAST
CONNECTION
COOKBOOK

A Guide to Good
Nutrition and Better Health

A Companion to
"The Yeast Connection and the Woman"
and
"The Yeast Connection Handbook"

William G. Crook, M.D.
&
Marjorie Hurt Jones, R.N.

TIRED-
SO TIRED
and the
"yeast
connection"

WILLIAM G. CROOK, M.D.

with a foreword by Bernard Rimland, Ph.D., Director, Autism Research Institute

I hope you'll like this book. And even if you don't I'd love to hear from you. Please send me your comments by mail, fax or e-mail. As a token of my appreciation, I'll send you a copy of one of my illustrated booklets.

- *Dr. Crook Discusses . . . Yeasts . . . and How They Can Make You Sick* (48 pages)
- *Dr. Crook Discusses Alternatives to. . . Ritalin . . . in the Management of ADHD* (32 pages)
- *You and Allergy* (32 pages)

Fax: 731-660-5029
E-mail: Wgcrook913@aol.com
Mail: P.O. Box 3246, Jackson, TN 38303

When you send me your comments, let me know which booklet you want, *Yeast, Ritalin* or *Allergy.*

William G. "Billy" Crook

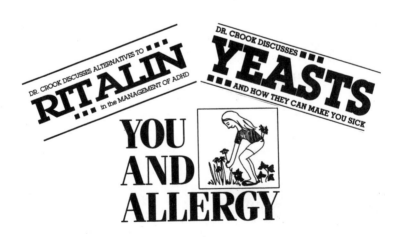